Manuela Heider de Jahnsen, MSc in Ayurveda, has studied Oriental Medicine since 1980. Studying the ancient systems of healing and putting them into practice allowed her to meet and work intensely with people from very different cultures and backgrounds, close and abroad. Through projects for the European Union, she got involved in integration plans for refugees and created intercultural care options for children in hospices.

She runs a clinic for Ayurveda, yoga therapy and acupuncture in Berlin, Germany, specialising in breathing explorations and workshops on the above themes worldwide, focusing on trauma. She is a free diver and uses water as an integrated part of treatments. She is a regular speaker in India.

Manuela Heider de Jahnsen, MSc

THE BREATH THAT MOVES INSIDE YOU

Dealing with Trauma-an Ayurvedic perspective

AUSTIN MACAULEY PUBLISHERS™

LONDON * CAMBRIDGE * NEW YORK * SHARJAH

A CIP catalogue record for this title is available from the British Library.

ISBN 9781398433380 (Paperback)
ISBN 9781398435209 (ePub e-book)

www.austinmacauley.co.uk

First Published 2024
Austin Macauley Publishers Ltd®
1 Canada Square
Canary Wharf
London
E14 5AA

To my grandchildren, Livi and Bela, and all the children of the world who inherit the planet and the knowledge from all of us. Let's thrive for the best.

This work is dedicated to the unconditional love received from my daughters, Naira, Mimi and Elliot. Despite me coming home late every night; too late for their little lives. Taking full responsibility, I was carried away by the miracles of sadness, grief, surviving and healing. I love nothing more in this world than these three wonderfully strong and independent women, who say I inspire them to be passionate about what one does.

As the saying goes, "If one does what one loves, one never works a single day in life." Their belief in the world as a safe place was something I thrived for, yet sometimes failed miserably. However, they always motivated me through their words and ideas of love, gender and revolution. Regardless of some disputable choices, most turned out well-thought and eventually became enjoyable self-inquiry projects leading towards a successful and happy life.

This book is, of course, dedicated to my fabulous teachers and Gurujis in Ayurveda:

First, Vaidya S.N. Gupta from P.D. Patel Ayurveda Hospital, J.S. Ayurveda Mahavidyalaya, Nadiad, Gujarat, India, who always answered when I doubted, "Try!" One can only wish for the support, confidence and guidance he has given! I thank him for having me as a regular speaker at the International Ayurveda Conferences in Nadiad, Gujarat, organised by the same Institute. So much gratitude.

My two loved and adored professors and vaidyas, Ram Manohar and Martin Mittwede, who have been gently guiding me through all rafts and preventing me from falling into the potholes of wrong assumptions or cultural appropriation.

Vaidya Prof. Ram Manohar, Amrita School of Ayurveda, *Kollam*, *Kerala*, India, whom I thank sincerely from my heart for accepting me as his student. At the time I started my book, I was partially blind. My papers were a mess and he just said, "I would love to read more!"

Thanks to him for the sheer confidence he re-established, so I could finally make it! Thanks for helicoptering me! And still seeing me!

Professor Martin Mittwede, Germany, for his kindness and strong support of wild ideas, for being my inspirational mentor and never short on best advice. There are so many more family, friends and assistants over my 45 years of practice that should all be named and thanked, but there is not enough space on paper however, an endless list of gratitude.

To all my friends and family here and in India who contributed in many different ways: Helga Heider, my mother, Gisela Borras, my auntie, Sanjay Sharma and his entire family, Kamal, Dimpy and Pamela Sharma and my aunties and uncles Sharma, Deepak Barthwal, Deepak, the astrologer, Maha Devdas and—

Elmar Stapelfeldt, for challenging my taste buds with his famous *dravya guna* introduction! Without him, all my studies would have lacked bite and taste!

Surinder Singh, Rishikesh. He is my most beloved yoga teacher of all time. I sat with him for twenty years, still wondering how it is possible to be so loving and kind. He allowed me to see a pure *sattvic* mind.

Giovanni Frazzetto, whose exploration in the art and science of intimacy and relationship, love and family, has always been a long discussion and cultural inquiry (with almost no—coffee).

Bettina Schuler from Citizen2Be, for allowing me to share her views and work with the most amazing Syrian refugee project I know.

Kerstin and Mark Rosenberg, founder of The Rosenberg Akademie, Birstein— Europe's biggest Ayurveda and Yoga Academy. They created a place of learning, studying, connection and excellence from which I could always start fresh, feel inspired and stay connected to my Indian roots. I am so grateful to be a teacher and lecturer at the Ayurveda Yoga Chikitsa Department and a speaker at the regularly held Symposium in Birstein.

To my friends who became assistants and assistants who became friends, without whom I would not have accomplished so much:

Bnaya Halperin-Kaddari, a special thanks for exploring *the heart's prana, sound and soul connection*. Without him and his curiosity, the deep dive would not have been possible.

Dr Anastasia Shchedrina, my other "Ayurveda-half" and "Ocean sister", exploring the wonder oils of life and friendship: *abhyanga* means "love"; indeed the second best *abhyanga* therapist in the world (the first one I have not met yet).

Beate Friede, a kind soul at my side for thirty continuous years of deep yoga practice, acupuncture training and deep friendship without boundaries. Pure trust and playfulness.

Masami Kurihara, for our famous silent communication with her deep understanding and practice of loving-kindness and deep yoga.

Romi Deift, for the beauty of precision in style and numbers, pure *pranayama*— diamond-cut.

Magda Torres, for grace and day-glow to the yoga artwork and therapy of mindfulness in a jaguar style.

Yuri Kadzman, for a constant inspirational quest for truth; heart and mind can be one until it gets separated for a question.

Christopher Farrugia, adding taste to healing.

Endless thanks to these remarkable friends for the study:
Sueno, the great loss.

Kapil Malhotra, the open wounded and healing soul of the Taj.

Namic Macik, the light in the darkness of fire.

Ashkan Sepahvand, the radiating galaxy that always turns back home.

Jasmin Kokkola, the forest, moss and the lake of honesty.

Sejla Pierrot, close to the heart, always.

Gerda Klingenböck, the guardian angel with a golden heart and ghee, living in the forest.

Jadi Carboni, the graceful dancer through life's music.

Sooki Raffael, whose love for life was like the breath itself.

Natasha Ginwala, for adding the subtleness and cultural responsibility.

Catrina Armendariz, for a fresh outlook on the next project, her courage and open-mindedness.

To the trust and faith that my patients have in me. They were ready to open their wound again for contributing to the healing of many.

Special thanks to Milena Kremakova and Farisa Sepahvand for hours of patient editing and dedicated blind support from the heart!

Berlin, Germany, 2023

"As human beings, we have a penchant to connect. Like waves cling to shore, so we are inclined to attach. There may be seasons of low tide, an occasional desire to drift solo, or storms that strand us, but eventually we will seek or return to a harbour. Loneliness can kill, while togetherness revives."

Giovanni Frazzetto

Is it a gift having survived trauma oneself, having grown into the understanding of recovery and healing? As one patient said, "I would not call it a gift, as I don't want to give it to anyone else."

From there on, I decided to pass on my knowledge of healing.

Foreword

I have known Manuela Heider de Jahnsen as a compassionate practitioner of Yoga therapy in Germany and a passionate student of Ayurveda. Over the years, she has evolved into a skilled therapist offering solace to mentally traumatised patients. She also words with people suffering from addictions. It was no surprise to me that she was inspired to apply the knowledge she gained from Ayurveda to benefit her patients.

Post-traumatic stress disorder (PTSD) is a debilitating mental disorder prevalent worldwide, affecting people of any ethnicity, nationality or culture. A deeply threatening or scary event can trigger this mental condition and though effective treatments are available, the patients experience much pain during recovery.

As a result of scholarly engagement with the classical ayurvedic texts and interaction with Ayurveda clinicians and her insights, Manuela has developed an ayurvedic narrative of PTSD as a type of extrinsic unmāda (mental disorder). Classification and description of the stages in Trauma experience based on the dosa response to the trauma from an ayurvedic perspective is a clinically helpful framework to fine-tune the treatment based on ayurvedic principles and maximise the outcomes.

A vibrant and diverse collection of patient case studies illustrate the practical benefits of her integrative approach of combining yoga and ayurvedic with the modern medical understanding of PTSD.

Manuela has painstakingly put together her clinical experiences in managing PTSD in her patients and stitched a very interesting framework for integrative therapy to fulfil the requirements of the Master's Program in Ayurveda at Rosenberg's European Academy of Ayurveda, Birstein, Germany.

She was ably guided by Prof. Martin Mittwede, who oversees the Master's Program in Ayurveda that is validated by Middlesex University, UK.

It was an engaging experience for me to co-guide Manuela during her thesis word. I am sure her thesis will open new avenues for integrating Ayurveda, Yoga and Modern Medicine into novel approaches to improving mental health. The fact that Manuela's word is based on actual clinician patient encounters supports her insights and discussions with an experiential backdrop that would be extremely valuable for clinicians and researchers in the field.

With Yoga, Ayurveda and Modern Medicine integrated into a comprehensive treatment program, Manuela addresses the human being in totality and give attention to the individual's soul, mind and body.

Vaidya Ram Manohar is an Ayurveda physician based in India and heads Research in Ayurveda at Amrita Vishwa Vidyapeetham, ranked first amongst the private Universities of India. He has a particular interest in ancient Indian psychology and its clinical applications.

Prof. Ram Manohar

Ayurveda is a comprehensive traditional health and medical system that originated in ancient India over 2500 years ago. Yoga can be described as a path of self-awareness and self-knowledge that is meant to lead to an inner clear wisdom-filled realisation. With its application of meditative, breath—and body-related methods, it has numerous therapeutic implications.

In western reception, these two actually independent traditions have sometimes become mixed, so that the contours of the two systems do not always emerge clearly. In therapeutic work, however, ayurveda and yoga can enter into fruitful symbioses and complement each other.

Manuela Heider de Jahnsen is one of the pioneers of yoga therapy in Germany. In her decades of working with patients, she has not only built up a wealth of experience but also a special expertise in dealing with traumatised patients and those affected by addictions.

She accompanies these patients not only with a great deal of empathy, commitment and human attention, but also enables them to gradually regain contact with themselves through meaningful combinations of yogic exercises with ayurvedic therapeutic measures.

In both groups of patients or in the combination of the disorders, the inner centre of life is not seldom lost. Dissociative gaps open up between the psychic activities and the physical sensitivities. The separated dynamics provide for a variety of symptoms, such as anxiety, depressive episodes up to psychotic states.

Manuela successfully completed her studies in ayurvedic medicine under my supervision and wrote a master's thesis on the above-mentioned topic. In it, she reflects on the ayurvedic and western view of the clinical symptomatology and probes the various therapeutic approaches in a systematic overview.

A central core of the work is the carefully elaborated and touching case documentations, in which the therapy strategies and the underlying rationale are described in an exemplary way. In this way, the reader gains an insight into "work in progress" and can develop therapeutic paths for severely burdened patients through his or her own reflection.

In this sense I wish the work an attentive readership, which opens the possibility to comprehend holistic and individually adjusted therapy ways. The spiritual dimension is not to be disregarded. However, this does not come in a dogmatic form, but is oriented toward the reality of the patient's life.

Of fundamental importance is the question of how the loose ends of life can be put back together, how a person can regain the courage to look forward and find his or her own way into a lost space of freedom.

Prof. Dr Martin Mittwede habilitated with a research project on Ayurveda medicine at the Goethe University Frankfurt am Main. He directs a master's program in which physicians and other medical professionals are trained in ayurvedic medicine at an academic level. He has published numerous books and professional publications on the topics of Ayurveda, yoga and Asian philosophy.

In his psychotherapeutic practice, Prof. Mittwede combines holistic approaches of humanistic and analytical psychology with mindfulness, meditation and spirituality.

Contact:
www.mittwede.net
dr.mittwede@t-online.de
0049 176 24159749

Manuela has always taught me to be curious. Her interests are extremely broad and she is open to everything—that is, everything which she can use to help her patients. She has been active in the field of naturopathy for more than 40 years. This book embodies Manuela's professional journey as a naturopathy practitioner, conceptualised through an academic, scientific lens.

For the past years, ayurveda and yoga have been the main systems within which Manuela has been working; she has chosen to treat trauma and PTSD using the two systems. Ayurveda puts much emphasis on the need for balance and her book is also about balance between western and eastern medical systems; between science and intuition; between critical thinking and faith.

Manuela herself admits to being of mixed descent, as well as to having been connected to Asia since her childhood. This is clearly reflected in her book, as she treats yoga and ayurveda with great respect, avoiding both the western colonial approach and an unreasonable fascination for the two systems. Manuela's book discusses the phenomenon of trauma and PTSD as well as standard psychotherapy methods from unexpected angles.

For instance, she uses her own example to illustrate that trauma may result in a seemingly 'normal' behaviour such as an ideally clean house or any other type of extreme perfectionism—something to which the western therapeutic school pays little attention. Of great interest are her reflections on memory and reminiscences, e.g., on how patients get tired of having to turn to their reminiscences frequently.

Thus, the corporal approaches and the ancient knowledge offered by ayurveda and yoga can prove highly effective in treating trauma and handling PTSD. The classification of stages of PTSD based on the doshas and gunas dominant at each stage, along with the ensuing therapeutic recommendations, has particularly fascinated me, as this is the first time I encounter such an approach. Notably, these are not mere ideas or hypotheses—these are the results of Manuela's extensive empirical research.

The author pays particular attention to the issues facing women in modern society, including the violence they have to endure—something that is still frequently silenced. Most notably, Manuela always respects her patients' cultural identities and backgrounds and she considers those factors during therapy.

Of course, this has been reflected in the book as well. Detailed descriptions of yoga breathing exercises and ayurvedic procedures showcase the author's professionalism, but they also speak volumes about how she has been transferring the knowledge provided under the two Indian systems into the western one.

The book will be of interest to a wide range of readers because it significantly broadens one's perceptions of trauma and PTSD, providing unexpected perspectives on those issues.

Therapists will be interested in this book because it gives an account of the author's unique, years-long experience in naturopathy, conceptualised academically within the context of the western medicine. As for me, I am endlessly grateful for having Manuela in my life; for the many years of joint work; for the fact that she has become my friend and mentor; for how she discovers the untapped potential in her friends and colleagues and helps them harness it.

We have been working together for many years now and I still learn something new from Manuela—not just in terms of Ayurveda, but also in terms of the sheer curiosity about the various aspects of life, the desire to try them out—and then to offer the best to patients!

Dr Anastasia Shchedrina

Introduction to the Discussion of Trauma and Intercultural Dialogue

An Overview

Trauma is part of life. Nasty things happen to us, loved ones die, we lose and win and lose again; we suffer from unexpected illnesses, assault, accidents and so we all will be experiencing the pain of losing loved ones. However, some of us might come out of it and live even better or meaningful lives while others struggle and don't blossom. In this book, I will try to shed light on options to end the frozen time, the burnouts, the stormy rocky times of victims' narratives.

The Traumatised Self

Trauma, a psychological impact, has reached the daily lives of everyone as a term for describing the aftermath of shock, grief and terror. However, in contrast to the common knowledge of the word, understanding victims and their individual needs, reactions and adaptations are far from it. Nevertheless, victims have to live with a stigma. It ranges from provoking an assault or attack, "getting over it," "it was not that bad," or they were "weak" personalities anyhow.

Stigmatisation of victims and disbelief are often causing more harm in the long term than the traumatising situation itself by creating repression. *These strategies, which consume significant cognitive resources, have been associated with negative effects on interpersonal, physiological and emotional functioning (—)* (Trauma Therapy in Context, 2012).

The victim becomes imprisoned in shame, guilt and denial. For recovery, stepping out of the shame trap seems to be an essential first step to self-care and responsibility for further actions.

Trauma induces constant distress to the body and the mind, most likely reducing decision-making abilities, sleep, good health and long life. The various ways the victim adapts to the constant stress often include self-harm and risky behaviour, commonly associated with substance abuse, eating disorders, violence or depression. Suicide is sometimes the only way for the victim to escape the pain.

To induce self-care, modify the stress response and initiate self-healing processes, therapists become challenged with multiple reactions to the same stress factors of trauma. To develop successful treatments, they react differently, with significant differences in cultures, personalities, circumstances, repetition, single trauma, co-dependency, addiction, self-harm and violence. While the treatments are numerous, very little research is done to understand how and why patients respond to which type of intervention.

The base for the new data published in this book is my practice Society of Friends, a small clinic for complementary medicine and naturopathy in the centre of Berlin.

As the founder and head of the clinic for the last 40 years, my clinic developed complementary and alternative treatment schemes and solutions for traumatised patients. A group of assistants, apprentices, friends and students constantly accompanied, contributed and observed the treatments, but the best help came from the patients themselves. Since starting from scratch, I came across patients with unexpected troubling or paradox reactions to regular Ayurveda therapies.

Intense studies on trauma followed, from the recent research publications in the western hemisphere, classical Chinese and Japanese medicine, to ayurvedic scriptures and yoga texts concerning the topic. The topic, in respect, what it could have been in the ancient scriptures of other cultures. However, encouraged through my professors I developed a scheme of interpreting symptoms and factors in relation to therapies.

This foundation developed a unique classification of the patient's individual needs and strengths. With this information, there is the possibility to optimise Trauma and PTSD (Post Traumatic Stress Disorder) treatments through a simple symptom related tables in relation to the Ayurveda Dosha system. This system is developed out of hundreds of patients' experiences in my clinic and published here for the first time. The traditional Ayurveda treatment plans evaluated are suitable for modern patients.

However, the main question had to be asked initially:

Is it possible to authentically adopt medical systems, understandings and beliefs from other cultures?

And, how do we discover the differences when they might as well remain invisible to an observer whose thought process is shaped by their own culture? A common problem of intercultural studies is, assuming to understand what the other speaker is talking about, thus missing out on crucial cultural differences. In the words of a Korean feminist translator of Walter Benjamin:

Translation is a Mode= Translation is an Anti-neo-colonial Mode. She states *"re-translation" or "racial-hybrid" as a conclusion of all translation attempts. A form, a mode. This productive tension (a possible mistranslation?) indicates a formative activity simultaneous to the occupation of translation's modality: an incorporeal material, language trans-forms, re-forms, con-forms, de-forms.* (Ashkan Sepahvand, 2020)

Is it possible to penetrate high complexity beliefs and insights from other cultures? Below we try to ask, analyse the methodic views and present a holistic approach that highlights the eastern and western ways to integrate modern trauma therapy concepts, evaluate and use them in a holistic context of Ayurveda.

Is it possible to reveal and discover one's assumptions, beliefs and convictions as unconfirmed concepts?

Is it possible to integrate different ways of thinking into dominant western thinking, in which consciousness, unconsciousness and matter play an entirely different role in the complexity of a human being? Is it possible to see the individual's health separately from the health of the environment, the ocean and the planet as a whole? Ayurveda imposes the duty to dedicate and contribute to universal factors such as *dharma* as a duty.

How do we use western medicinal research within systems in which healing is more than healing of the mind or the body, but always of a mind-body continuum, as there is no natural separation between those? This work dedicates to finding those answers.

Complex systems of philosophical inquiries enrich the cultural beliefs in western culture through trade and exchange for thousands of years. However, the Jewish-Christian-Cartesian cultural heritage carries out one of the significant differences in western view towards eastern conception: the duality of mind and body. An aspect of Ayurveda is majorly vital for this thesis; Ayurveda has no psychology, only psychiatry.

As Professor Ram Manohar (Amrita College, Kollam Kerala) states: *"The mind can only be studied separately when it is insane.* From an ayurvedic perspective, the body and mind are one single continuum. *Like a vessel and ghee, they are interconnected* as Vaidya Ram Manohar says: *Looking at things that are the same like hot and cold—they are related as a continuum, that keeps on influencing every other point on the continuum."* (Ram Manohar, 2012)

A synthetic philosophical approach like Ayurveda can integrate an analytical approach, like western psychology, nutrition, etc. However, the western biomedical approach to health is analytical, non-holistic, dualistic and therefore disabled to integrate a complex system like Ayurveda.

The Mind can only think of what is already known. Ludwig Wittgenstein states in his book *Tractatus Logicus Philosophicus*, that we can only ask questions of which the answers are known. Even if a particular thought could appear ground-breaking or out of the box, it is only a product of the limitation of human and, in particular cultural, thinking works.

Therefore, ayurveda and yoga could represent a way of bridging western and eastern therapeutic measures and thinking. Ayurveda and yoga are empirical sciences with the knowledge that can be experienced and observed. It is inductive-synthetic. However, both can be seen as inter-cultural empiric sciences because their science of experience and the applied methods are sensational and not limited to a particular country, belief, concept or paradigm. Experience is bound to the concept of experiencing and can only come through diligent practice.

Uniting and Dividing

Different cultures are different only to a certain extent. There is always an overlap of content, as all human beings share the same dreams and fears. Ultimately, similarities become overseen when focusing on differences. Differences become missed by focusing on similarities. Both options will not serve the purpose.

Instead, a middle ground must exist; a clear and respectful open dialogue. Beginning a profound, meaningful and constructive discussion is necessary to clarify terms and context. By *translating* singular words out of context, the translation cannot reflect the whole possible meaning. Meaning depends on context, story, background, history and the speaker and listener. Interpreting is the interaction of the speaker and the listener. *Interpreting* words instead helps to understand the experience and brings words into life.

Some words are kept in their original language to avoid misinterpretation. The original words clarify and classify the topic without discourse. The actual terminology in Sanskrit allows a deep inspection of the meaning of Ayurveda and the practice and philosophy of yoga. Although not all texts have been published in Sanskrit, it is the primary source language used in this thesis.

Simplifying and mixing concepts from different traditions can induce misleading assumptions. Clarifying terms and concepts are crucial to start a deep and meaningful dialogue between cultures to realise ideas and goals.

Eastern mind and medicine are based on an empirical and philosophical approach toward life, death, health, happiness and the mind's function. Empirical wisdom has been generated and collected over thousands of years, including countless case studies displaying success and failure.

Although Empirical knowledge is not ideological, it serves no other than the patient's interest. Over long periods, if a system becomes inefficient, it simply disappears. Ayurveda and yoga are collections of wisdom and philosophy spanning several millennia. The effectiveness of ancient systems of knowledge and practice, such as ayurveda and yoga, is proved by their continued existence.

In the sciences and concepts of yoga and ayurveda, the function of the mind—body—continuum is revealed in clear terms and with practical guidance. Empirical knowledge and hundreds of techniques for self-inquiry are present. Physical exercise (*asana*) and deep meditation (*dhyana*), breathing (*pranayama*), daily routine (*dinacharya*) and detailed description of the cause and effect of thoughts and actions *(karma)* are structured and explained. Nutrition and lifestyle (*ahara* and *vihara)* are the pillars of a system of rules and ethics that follow philosophical outlines. It follows the newer discoveries of the biorhythm of hormones and physiological changes.

Unlike western analytical philosophies that analyse particles and elements to explore the entire object, eastern philosophical traditions follow a so-called synthetic tradition that tries to understand form and function from wholeness.

The meaning of the word yoga is often translated as "unity, connection," while Ayurveda translates as "the science of life and death". Both ayurveda and yoga are different from western philosophies regarding their definition of time and space. Western concepts define a linear concept of time and space. While most eastern philosophies, ayurveda and yoga in particular, state a cyclic and rhythmic existence in which mind and matter repeatedly reoccur in the same way as the seasons of the year come and go (*samsara*).

The countless number of contradicting philosophies of India have not disappeared in modern days, nor have they been replaced by historical influences like imperialism or colonialism. Today, India has a broad spectrum of actively practiced beliefs and philosophies, from mono—to pantheism, tantrism and atheism.

As a social experience of diversity, innumerable beliefs and traditional rituals are described. Having a population of 3.5 billion people, India is woven together as a system of tolerance and diversity, often haunted by shadows of the opposite. Intolerance and even fanatism are the other sides of the historical multi-ethnic subcontinent. The philosophical and medical experiences and beliefs are joined together in Ayurveda, *Unani* and *Siddha* medicine (including tribal medical shamanic systems) in various yogic traditions like *Bhakti Yoga, Karma Yoga, Raja* Yoga and Tantric Yoga.

This picture reflects and incorporates the multiple changes in society (better to use the term—*societies* within the Indian subcontinent, not to mention the later division in India, Pakistan and Bangladesh) through invaders, natural disasters and the golden age within a historical timeline from the ancient past to the present day. It accepts and integrates traditions from the highest university standards with lab tests to procedures that summarise under the name of Shamanism, from *Rasaushadhis* (refining of toxic substances to eliminate toxicity) to reciting mantras, from touch and massage therapy to sexual practices in therapy.

According to the rituals of each belief and the *shastras*, it is possible to renounce the world or wholly embrace it, allowing everything to integrate into life and meaning. The sources of knowledge stretch from the high altitude of the Himalayas of Jammu and Kashmir to other Oriental traditions, like Tibetan, Mongolian and traditional Chinese medicine, all the way down to the damp swampy areas and deep green jungles of Kerala and Karnataka.

It covers knowledge of medical plants and traditions from the vast deserts of Rajasthan and those from agricultural settlements. It integrates the cow-based medicine of Uttar Pradesh with coconut oil preparations from Sri Lanka. The inner times within India range from cultures still in stone age manners in the forests of remote islands to rocket technology and the atomic power plants alongside the country. It covers most different medical traditions of a landmass that includes almost 1,500 official languages and about the same number of presumed languages and dialects with all their knowledge and practice.

There is a shared sense of analytical observation in modern biomedicine or western medicine. It includes the knowledge of germs as a paradigm and sets standards through dissection and laboratory measures. Western and modern medicine will establish a new standard when the old becomes outdated. Biomedicine represents the Cartesian belief that mind and body are separated. Biomedicine only dates back to the 19th century, marked by the invention of vaccines and the discovery of germs.

In comparison to Ayurveda's holistic view, it uses a database of analytics and measurements to quantify disease and the cell healing process. However, very little is known of the patient's recovery options and their self-healing ability, stamina, resilience options and so forth or even prevention through nutritional lifestyle components from stress reduction. Some GPs (General Practitioners) agree to psychosomatic sources of certain diseases. Organic disfunction and failure do not necessarily include better treatment options.

Modern psychological approaches towards disease often blame the patient. They are inefficient. *The view of sickness and death as a personal failure is a particularly unfortunate form of blaming the victim.* (When the body says No, Exploring the Stress disease Connection.) (Gabor Mate, 2011)

Mate is convinced that stress is most likely be transmuted into illness as it is a complicated cascade in our system that responds with physical and biochemical changes. Emotions are therefore able to change the function of hormonal glands, organs, oxygen supply, our whole way of thinking and responding to stressful situations.

Over time, our immune systems that was designed to protect us can turn against us. Gabor Mate lays down all the specific measures of how western biomedicine looks at all the details. In opposed to, Ayurveda looks at the whole. Ayurveda does not even end there: it expands its knowledge of the person by framing them into all interrelated connections of social relations, food, climate, age, the emotional state, the stars, whatever affects individual life in the endless web of creation.

Holistic medical approaches, such as Ayurveda, oppose medical experts' processes in one or two medical fields.

Integrating Ayurveda into a concept that reduces complex systems to the analytical separation of causes is most likely to fail.

Focusing on the treatment of the individual and providing complex structured multi-dimensional treatment plans, using the knowledge of analytics, could bring these two worlds together for the benefit of the patient. Respectfully, the knowledge of life and death (Ayurveda, Prof. Ram Manohar) and the inquiries into consciousness (yoga) should be carefully examined to understand recovery, resilience and healing in a holistic rather than in a reductionist way: B*ody and mind are one continuum* (Ram Manohar, Indic Studies*).*

When it comes to trauma, PTS (Post Traumatic Stress) and PTSD, the analysis of the differences in the definitions of mental health, mind and body and western trauma psychology is essential.

This book aims to inquire whether Yoga and Ayurveda provide suitable methodological approaches to diagnosing and treating trauma in an individually tailored treatment plan. It starts from the assumption that grief, sadness, anxiety, pain and fear are unavoidable and an integral part of life.

Why do human beings take different times to recover from trauma? Some individuals appear to recover quickly, while others recover only after a prolonged time or even not at all. It is to prove here that the complex socio-psycho-philosophical system of Ayurveda provides answers. Persisting socio-psychological and even physiological changes can be considered adaptation to the deep pain experienced.

In general, speaking about trauma is primarily about the adaption of trauma. Adaption is an uncomfortable way of living by avoiding unwanted memories. In the beginning, it feels comfortable as the avoidance of emotionally loaded memories reduces stress, but healing from traumatic injury is not taking place.

Further, structured avoidance plans for the patient need more strategic behaviour that will consume awareness and energy. The patient is not getting any closer to recovery through avoidance. Distress and psycho-physiological changes in the person lead to various patterns of avoidance. These patterns occur as well in PTS and PTSD.

However, some patients seem to not experience any distress at all, recover quickly or show other signs of successfully coping with the survival of trauma. It is crucial to understand why and how certain people develop better strategies for integrating the past into their narrative.

Ayurveda can provide answers by detailed predicting schemes of possible reactions of certain personality types, called *dosha* types. After intensive years of study, Society of Friends laid out tables of behaviour, responsiveness and adaption that allow the therapist to decide the best treatment more efficiently. At the same time, the research explicitly analyses some of the required treatment methods from Ayurveda and Yoga, *shirodhara* and *pranayama* and explains the proper use.

A change is needed, as both trauma victims and therapists long for solutions in the classical psychiatric treatments—an overload of patients with unwanted side effects, often without a long-term solution. Psychotherapy usually ends too early, as health insurance providers often refuse further payment when the patient is not recovering or is not responding to the particular method.

The example of the number in the *Chapter: Case Studies* will illustrate the impact of social insurance on recovery. What often remains uncleared is healing from trauma, as the acceptance and adaption to a chaotic world, a messy lifestyle or an unhappy relationship cannot be considered a sign of a healthy mental state. Adapting through therapy to an unhealthy and devaluating, disrespectful and toxic environment is not a sign of recovery.

Could the inability to accept and adapt to circumstances in which the person is living actually be a sign of mental recovery?

Many Trauma survivors already disguise themselves in so-called "normal" behaviour. They often disappear in a camouflaged, norm-filled and adapted lifestyle. Many of them are even over-achievers and develop symptoms like Compulsive Behaviour Disorders. The deep pain often remains undetected as an always "spotless house," a "very busy-late-night-still-working-mum," and the "extra busy school kid" are society role models of success.

It can take years until the tragedy behind those norm-over-fulfilling behaviour might unravel as an adaption, as a way to explain the lack of friends and intimacy ("too busy!"), as a measure to try and keep life under control. Drug addicts, patients with eating disorders and those with Compulsive Behaviour

Disorder report that their behaviour gave them a sense of control. Living has turned into a function as opposed to an experience.

Meaning in Life: Positive "side effects" of Holistic Treatment with Ayurveda:

An important focus in Ayurveda is meaning-making. Meaning-making had become a vital tool in the treatment of Society of Friends, although there was no initial planned redirecting towards meaning in life. A purpose in life seemed to have been a side effect of successful treatment. Patients reported a change of attitude and an increasing duration of experiencing satisfaction or happiness.

It is the key that through meaning making the person is able to step out of the anxious preoccupation of repeating the traumatic event over and over, by adjusting and integrating experiences and move away from it by doing so. This explains the effects of our treatments that are rooted in complex philosophical and medical contexts coming from Ayurveda and yoga, but the research on achieving meaning-making is far from studied in the west.

However, it is a crucial tool of ayurvedic and yogic procedures. As quite a few patients were recovering from drug addiction, this aspect was essential. Any drug/alcohol addiction or other addictive behaviour (shopping, cutting, gambling, sex, food, etc.) leads to momentary relief from unpleasant emotions. It pilots patients to sudden changes in their emotional state (high or peak).

It was complicated in the past (before ayurvedic and yoga treatment existed at the clinic) to communicate otherwise. A life without substance addiction is not necessarily experienced as more of a "high" life but mostly just a life without substance abuse, without the dopamine rush as a reward without bliss or ecstasy.

Instead, the user may experience reduced dissociation and improvement of self-control of emotions, effects and distress reduction. Experiences of deep contentment can bridge the brains need for peak experiences where it allows us to create a feeling of being part of a larger community or feeling connected to the whole. These feelings are described as being in harmony and from this place, only creativity in exploring life in a free mind can occur.

This is very different to the encounter of generated peak experiences through drugs, partying or business success, where a not a constant repetition of these experiences is required, but they also fade over time and have to be continuously topped up. Here we are describing again the way to addiction.

Ayurveda might reconstruct feelings inherited by the (healthy) child: mindfulness and meaning.

A meaningful life provides us with the nourishment of the experience of the here and now, where we experience the present moment and embracing it. Breathing, oiling, human connections, love allow us to feel grounded in an increased attention to sensations, thoughts, emotions and physical sensations. The book will present my studies over the last forty years to answer whether ayurveda and yoga can perhaps provide the qualities for healing and the procedures conducted for the western patient living in a modern world to a wider audience.

Trauma—A Brief Overview of the Recent Research in Western Countries

The globalised dimension of war, assault, natural disasters and diseases created a growing awareness of the traumatic incidents and their often lifelong damaging character. The Austrian society for "Traumafolgestörungen" has declared that focus has been very much on the individual that sufferes from trauma, less on the socio-culturalcontext.

In a psychological context, the term Trauma describes an unexpected, sudden event of significant threat. Repetition of traumatic incidents often occurs. The events cause serious extreme stress responses in the body and mind, often with feelings of fear of death, panic and helplessness. It does not describe the aftermath, adaptation, survival, coping mechanisms, depressive mood disorders, ADH or ADHS and other related conditions.

A difference in diagnosis and treatment has to be made clear between the event of trauma and the possible aftermath, as Post-Traumatic Stress Disorder or Post Traumatic Depression.

Not all traumatic events lead necessarily to PTSD (Post Traumatic Stress Disorder).

As traumatic events are most likely to be experienced by every living being, PTSD is not.

PTSD is marked by:

- Intrusive memories of the traumatic event
- Systematic avoidance of all trauma-related aspects (dates, smells, locations, sounds, etc.)
- Cognitive symptoms of autonomic nervous hyperactivity

The diagnosis and treatment have become crucial in western countries, as trauma-related illnesses are relevant factors in the health system and an economic element.

The request for effective treatment is drastically rising.

Adverse changes in the personality, a decrease in cognitive functions and moods are significant markers for PTSD. Other characteristics include: dissociative disruption of memory, persistently negative assumptions about oneself or the world, shame and guilt or other negative emotional states, including depression, suicidal attempts, self-harming behaviour, anger and rage, loss of interest and significant decline of psycho-social participation, depersonalisation, derealisation and emotional numbness characterise the patients who suffered a traumatic event initially and developed later PTSD.

Complex PTSD patients show almost all mentioned signs, while in PTSD, the patient shows at least two to three characteristics of the above.

Physiological responses can include:

Blood pressure can vary from low to high, swings or an extreme amplitude in mm Hg (millimetre of mercury). Hypervigilance and insomnia increase the constant stress response in the body, leading to several psycho-somatic illnesses, like inflammations of the gut lining, tension headaches, chronic pain syndromes and most likely auto-immune diseases.

In cases of "complex PTSD," patients show a broad and complex set of symptoms. It often includes increased emotional dysregulation, chronic self-destruction, dissociative behaviour and somatic symptoms. Altered beliefs about the self and dysfunctional relationships are signs of complex PTSD. Prolonged mourning and grief are also a disorder based on PTSD.

Overview of symptoms of PTSD/Trauma According to the American Psychological Association

For a person to receive a diagnosis of PTSD, they must meet the criteria set out by the American Psychological Association's (APA) Diagnostic and Statistical Manual Fifth Edition (DSM-5).

According to these guidelines, the person must have been exposed to, including during professional duties or witnessing others to be exposed to death or threatened death, serious injury or sexual violence or during professional duties. If symptoms of distress, re-experiencing the trauma, images, etc., continue for more than a month, avoidance symptoms cause disruption of normal life and are affecting the mind and thinking process by repletion, hyperalert reactions, nightmares, sleeplessness or flashbacks the patient would be recognised with a PTS.

It is important to understand that flashbacks are not a proof of the distress as the human brain can also imagine events, but that the opposite can be also the truth: the patients' inability to remember anything of the traumatising event. This is not only the case for small children, but can be part of the patients' untold story at any age. Feelings of shame, guilt, self-blaming as well as difficulties in focusing on work, conversations, even TV programs can accompany the mental health problems like depression, phobias or anxiety disorders, to name only a few.

#Dr Gabor Mate sees a close pain connection through trauma to various mental health issues as well as Auto-Immune diseases like ALS, Rheumatoid diseases, Lupus, etc.

However, seeing dysfunctional relationships that are often trauma bond explains the tragedy that many patients find themselves in, by repeating traumatic incidents involuntarily, but by being unable to identify warning signs that a healthy individual would have realised much earlier.

Physical signs are not included in the recognition of victims of trauma, according to the psychiatric manual; however, they are the signs that patients carry for long and often are the cause that allow the patients to finally to seek help without admitting the emotional changes, the panic, the grief, the shame. Physical symptoms can also be the only hint of a forgotten story, to a denied place in the life of the victim.

Children are often acting out their traumatic experience through play, in drawings or that they display an overall adapted behaviour. The "good child", the always pleasing child, is a warning that teachers, kindergarten teachers or others involved should be noticing as an alarm sign. Bedwetting, obsession with electronic games, anxiety and isolation, aggression and irritability are signs that a society widely ignores as the easy child is the so called " normal"

Resilience, Recovery, Treatment and PTSD

Recovery or healing can be possible depending on the individuals exposed to trauma, their resilience, the time and intensity of exposure to the distress, the immediate help and other factors. An important example of these well-supported recovery measures is Kapil's story in Case Studies. The Taj Mahal Hotel supported them in their financial and emotional way of recovering from the beginning.

Quantitative studies show that people experience several traumatic events in their lifetime (Kate M. Scott et al., 2013). Most of these traumatic biographical events become silently part of their history and shape their character. They also define how the person will deal with distress in the future. Yet, some individuals develop post-traumatic stress (PTSD). PTSD can last up to several days, weeks or even a lifetime. It often remains untreated and the possible three outcomes can occur:

—*complete recovery,*
—*resilience or,*
—*the development of post-traumatic stress disorder or complex PTSD.*

Recovery is the complete restoration of the person's psychological and physiological health. It characterises complete remission of all signs of distress, such as anxiety, avoidance of places, smells, special occasions places, normal blood pressure (BP) and pulse frequency. Sleep and eating habits, as well as sexual function, are fully restored.

Resilience is the person's ability to restore and maintain equilibrium after the distress and handle triggering events with awareness of own reactions, such as the arousal of anxiety or the avoidance of places, people, occasions or smells. Sleep, eating habits and sexual function are restored gradually to a normal mode or are consciously controlled.

PTSD is a dysfunctional response to distress by developing depression, anxiety, sleep, eating disorders or the inability to perform an "average" sex life. It often characterises the avoidance of places, people, occasions or smells. A person with PTSD cannot control her response to reoccurring distress of the same kind or even other types. The mere retelling of the memorised traumatic event is often enough to cause arousal (see the definition of APA above).

Noteworthy are the latest publications from G. Mate. He states that the co-morbidity after trauma is like drug abuse and CBD (Compulsive Behaviour Disorder) signs of adaptation to constant stress, lighting different approaches in health care. If poly-toxicity is concerned with treating PTSD, the abusive addictive behaviour is treated before the PTSD.

If poly-toxicity is considered adaption, the treatment of PTSD would be more important as the adaptive behaviour would fade. Mate, In the Realm of the Hungry Ghosts (2018) and other papers and lectures reveal the patients' intensity to escape the memories by adapting to them. Aristotle called the memory a " stamp on running water".

Recent research shows the chances of being exposed to traumatic incidents in the US is 60% compared to Algeria's 90%. There is a significantly high number of intra-personal violence (gun violence) in the US while developing countries report trauma merely after natural disasters. Europe, though, shows very different numbers.

While in the US, 10% of women have lifelong PTSD and 5% of men (Norris and Slone, 2014). In Europe, the incidence is lower than 1,5%. It is essential to analyse these differences. A big part is the socio-psychological after-care in the US and Germany. A functioning health care system that provides aid in emergencies is undoubtedly an important factor in understanding recovery.

The situation for women worldwide is dramatic and mostly unspoken. Systematic rape during armed conflicts is considered a war crime but has hardly ever been respectfully treated. Each country fails to take responsibility and blames other countries for their problems. The numbers of domestic violence, rape and other physical or psychological assaults or even killing do not differ so much. What differs is more or less the way of carrying out violence against women, POCs (People of Colour) or the LGBTQ+ community.

The list of violence is long and includes rape within marriage or dating relationships or rape by strangers, unwanted sexual advances or sexual harassment, including demanding sex in return for favours. The cruelty towards children, particularly the mentally disabled and adults, is overwhelming and well-hidden.

In many countries, sexual violence and domestic violence are covered early by forced marriage or cohabitation, including child marriage. Denying the right to use contraception or to adopt other measures to protect against sexually transmitted diseases and forced abortion are violent acts against the sexual integrity of women. Female genital mutilation, including an inspection for virginity, interferes with human rights. Forced prostitution and trafficking of people for sexual exploitation are unfortunately not even the end of the list of cruelties.

Data on the Risk of Developing PTSD After Different Types of Impact and Experience

Being personally involved in a serious accident, suffering from a potentially deadly disease or surviving a serious injury, sexual assault or physical assault with or without injuries are the major causes of traumatic experiences, however, violence is mostly experienced by women and the LGTBQ+ community outside wars.

When the Past invades the present and leaks into the future

Memory alterations	Emotional changes and responses	Physical sensations	Relationship changes and issues
Concentrating for a short period without switching is possible, however, tasks that need longer focus are interrupted. Procrastination	Anxiety, anxious	High stress level reflects in hormonal changes	Hostility
Problems remembering aspects of the traumatic experience, the circumstances and details	Fear of resembling situations, avoidance of places, smells, sounds.	Physical exhaustion, fatigue	Withdrawal, feeling estranged
Decisions making fails because of inability to plan	Shock	Interrupted sleep, difficulty falling asleep, waking up during the night, urgent urination at night, early awakening	Reduced or no interest in sexual interaction
Mental or cognitive confusion, inability to follow instructions, rules, rhythms, regulations or provide daily routines	Grief, sadness, mourning that exceeds 6 weeks	Headaches, migraines, visual problems	Irregular or reduced work or school patterns
Painful memories of the event of the traumatic experience thoughts about what happened, how one could have reacted better, saved lives, etc.	Irritability, easily startled	Nausea, binge eating, anorexia and other emotional digestive problems	Blaming others, oneself
A sense of being lost, alone, losing visual control of the surrounding area, feeling disoriented	numb or detached feelings towards previous emotional meaningful situations, lack of happiness, joy, lack of physical	Increased heart beat rate up to 180 beats on arousal, increased or drastic decreased BP	A desire to hide, hibernate nest and avoid any contact with the world or social interactions

	sensations, whether pain or pleasure		
	Guilt, shame, vulnerability	light-headedness	Over-protectiveness (helicoptering)of family members whether involved in the trauma or absent
	Feelings of being alone, helpless, lost in space, abandoned	A temporary or consistent loss of interest in or pleasure from usual activities	
	Alienation with family and friends, as they signal, "it's time to get over it," vulnerable to toxic positivity: "look at the bright side, you are here now! Be happy. Others have more problems, etc."		
	A feeling of vulnerability to words, gestures, easily mislead or misinterpreted facial or emotional expressions of others		

A General Overview of Symptoms of PTSD/ Trauma and the Classification According to Neuro-Physiological and Psychological Symptoms in the Research of Society of Friends, Berlin, 1987-2020

Layout: Using the sources from Peter Levine and Bessel van der Kolk and the catalogues of psychiatry in the US and Germany. The tables reflect the research done at the Society of Friends. Some of the described symptoms overlap in two or more categories, yet the symptoms are placed where dominating aspects are found.

Neurological Symptoms	Physiological Symptoms	Psychological Symptoms
Sleep disorder: too little, interrupted or prolonged sleep time into the midday	*Chronic Pain Syndrome*: particularly neck, shoulders, back, pain in the chest (fake heart attack) increase of cortisol, prolactin	*Fear of* diseases, immobility, germs, people, dark, certain places, certain or all noises, fear of failure, fear of the end of the world
Nervousness, Irritability, Anxiety: change of brain response and activity in the emotional centre	Irritable Bowel Syndrome, indigestion, Diabetes Type 2, Insulin Intolerance Syndrome	Depression, Borderline Personality Disorder, hyper agility, euphoria, lack of hope
Forgetfulness, lack of memory of the event as well as loss of memory for daily needs	Heartbeat irregularity, increase of heartbeat to 220	Anorexia Nervosa, Bulimia, binge eating, suicidal
Digestive disorder as a response to increased activity of the sympathetic nervous system: hyperacidity, increasing under stress	Blood Pressure: secondary high BP, constantly too high, too low, too low or too big amplitude increase of cortisol, prolactin	Self—destructive or self-inhibiting behaviour: cutting, not allowing oneself to experience pleasure, not exercising or too much exercising, indulging in recreational drug(s), addiction of various kinds.
Learning difficulties, ADS (Acquired Demyelinating Syndrome), ADD	Cold sweat, profuse sweating	Constant high stress response, easily startled, easily disappointed
Dizziness, vertigo, tinnitus, shakiness	Breathing difficulties, wheezing	Feeling of loneliness, being overly pleasant or overly unpleasant in social behaviour, narcissistic

Overview of the Divergence of Study Groups Suffering Trauma and PTSD

Until now, the victims and survivors of trauma are not fully understood. What makes a survivor a victim and how long might the symptoms last? What are the generally agreed symptoms and what could be the individual's symptoms?

The answers will differ according to every psychiatric school. The incidents of individual symptoms are hardly recognised in relation to the complexity of a person as a whole, their surroundings, abilities and incapability before and after. A psychiatric condition or definition cannot reveal the individual's truth, beliefs, resilience or suffering. The true self cannot unleash from the point of view of pathology.

Instead, a person that has experienced severe and exceptional stress might bring everything with them to recover. This part of the individual, the healthy survival instinct, self-care, self-love, trust and faith, must be rediscovered, nourished and well-supported. It seems eager to develop a view of the person besides pathology, as the definition limits the patient's options for recovery.

Seeing the Differences—Understanding the Unity

Differences in recovery measures laid out by Bessel van der Kolk, Levine and others between soldiers and other survivors:

-the time frame in which the victim receives help

-social status after the attack

-financial support

-medical care

-availability of support groups

-family-related problems

These measures explain some of the differences in the diagnosis and treatment or even optional recovery on its own. An American veteran served the country, while a sex worker who experienced assault and rape will be most likely offended or even blamed for having the incident provoked. Therefore, not all data on trauma from American soldiers can apply to the current trauma and PTBS treatment in Europe or elsewhere.

A close look at the numbers of violence against women shows that worldwide at least every third woman is exposed to domestic violence, rape or other damaging violent experiences in the course of her life. Two out of every three people killed worldwide are women. In Germany, the numbers are not much different, with statistics reporting that at least one in every four women have been subjected to violence and rape in their lifetime (source: Ministry for Family, Seniors, Women and Youth,2019).

More than every day, women are domestically abused by their spouses. A woman gets killed by her spouse every other day. In total, 188 women were killed in 2019 alone by their partners in Germany. The "Agency for Equal Rights of the European Union" conducted the world's most considerable research on violence against women.

They discovered that 62 million women experienced physical or sexual violence and were assaulted after the age of 15 (33%) and that more than 41 million women experienced physical or sexual assault in their relationships (22%)More than half of the world's female population have been sexually assaulted (55%) and about a third of the confirmed cases end in reports that it had been professionally related men like their boss, colleague.

The numbers for LQTBQ+ are far higher however, in many countries they cannot come forward. Even the above numbers I would doubt, as I see more people as victims of sexual assault that have never reported their experience, being in fear of being judged, discriminated or facing rude behaviour, further assault or other painful newly traumatising situations at police stations. We can only imagine how big these numbers are in real life, as almost 70 % of all victims have not been reporting the assault to the police.

According to the statics of criminal assaults against women in Germany, published at Violence against Women, an EU-wide Survey, 2017 a number of 69.000 women suffering from direct physical assault, threat of physical assault around 16.700 (which clearly shows that even less women report threat, or, the threats have not been taken seriously and did not make it into the police records for various reasons. LGTBQ+ assaults are not yet listed specifically). Severe physical damage was reported in 11.800 cases and stalking, a forceful threat in another 2000 cases.

However, murder and killing of women in Germany in the year 2018 122 women were victims of femicide. Within relationships, 98 % of the victims of physical assault are women. Every hour a woman in Germany suffers from severe injuries inside her relationship.

A lot of further cases never get reported, as mentioned earlier and even if, fact is, that only 10-20% of rape cases in Germany end in a proper court case— and even more worrying, only in 8,4% of the final court cases the victim will win the case, often after years as mostly the evidence of rape within a relationship cannot be given easily. This still does not guarantee any compensation payment, treatment payment, care, protection or other help to not only survive the rape physically but emotionally.

The above examples of women's reality in Germany and other European countries societies lighten the fundamental problems in resourceful recovery options for non-veterans. Therefore, sensible investigations are necessary into the different sources, gender, POC (People of Colour), LGTBQ communities and refugee-related traumatisation to serve the patient's rights.

In my clinic we were very lucky that due to the location of the practice (close to yoga centres and big party places with high drug consumption) and my reputation in the field as well as involved in projects of the European union for the integration of refugees from Syria, Palestine and others that we saw hundreds of patients, that were from all cultural backgrounds, LGTBQ+, POC and were burdened with multiple traumatic experiences due to their background alone.

Left alone in a country with strict rules, a complicated language, different social support we often were the only place where they could help and support, connection and treatment. Waiting lists for trauma therapy easily exceed 3 years.

It is necessary to consider the multiple options of how a traumatic injury can occur and how it could or might unfold or end to understand trauma, PTSD and other related conditions. Studying and understanding the considerable differences of the individual to respond to specific traumatic triggers and how this could be controlled and finally, to research and understand how resilience, recovery and healing can take place. Data mainly deriving from soldiers with PTSD might mislead in the field.

Current Research on Trauma in the United States on Soldiers

Field studies in the US on trauma are extensively done on soldiers and veterans. These trauma patients display quite a standardised background in education, the details of the traumatising event and other socio-psychological parameters, according to demographic studies, like:

- Age (mostly between 19-45 years old)
- Sex (primarily men)
- Nationality (US American)
- Social status (legal job, hero of the country)
- Ethnicity (predominantly white)
- Religion (mostly Christians)

The number of Veterans with PTSD varies by service era. Examples are:

Iraq: 11-20% have been diagnosed with PTSD in a given year.
Vietnam War: 30% of Vietnam Veterans suffer PTSD in their lifetime other temporarily.

Other combat situations can add more stress to an already stressful situation. Contributing to PTSD and other mental health problems, these factors include what the person voluntarily did in the war, the politics around the war, where the battle is fought and the type of enemy the soldier had to face.

Another cause of PTSD in the military can be military sexual trauma (MST). MST is any sexual harassment or sexual assault that occurs while the person is in the military. MST can happen to both men and women and can occur during peacetime, training or war.

Among Veterans who use VA health care, about:

23 out of 100 women (or 23%) reported sexual assault when in the military.

55 out of 100 women (or 55%) and 38 out of 100 men (or 38%) have experienced sexual harassment in the military.

There are many more male Veterans than there are female Veterans. Interesting is the fact(that half of all Veterans with military sexual trauma are men.

Source: How common is PTSD in Veterans (2018)

A comparison to Trauma/PTSD patients in Europe and general study group of US-American soldiers might be difficult and not display the different needs as for my own study the following parameters were fact:

Trauma and PTSD, according to my studies at my clinic, had no preconditioning but other factors that made it more likely to happen.

we saw patients of:

- all ages
- primarily women and LQTBQ+
- Nationality (mostly European or Middle Eastern)
- Social status (all, but primarily low income, refugee status, single mothers, etc.)
- Ethnicity (diverse)
- Religion, diverse (Muslims, Jewish, Christians and others.)

Research on minority groups and race in the US highlights a society where even the research for treatment on trauma is predominantly done on white male Americans (There is a clear exception in the popular Trauma researcher Gabor Mate who's career as a physician involved predominantly first nation people with traumatic stress).

Therefore, the data might not be helpful to treat the majority of trauma victims who develop PTSD. In Europe, there is a multi-diversity of patients interested in more diverse backgrounds and a much lower number of veterans. The multi diversity of patients leads to a greater variety of treatment necessities. The studies focusing on one heterogenic group do not display the various backgrounds of traumatisation and the often-early onset of trauma. When it comes to aspects of building resilience and recovery, the data from US soldiers will not be helpful for the previously mentioned reason either.

Refugees in Europe

A vast number of traumatised people reached the shores of Europe in recent years as refugees from Syria, Ethiopia, Sudan and other countries. Worldwide an approximate of 25 Million people were leaving their countries, over half of them under the age of 18 and not all of them accompanied by their families.

The Convention in Geneva has claimed that a refugee is in "fear of being persecuted for reasons of race, religion, nationality, membership of a particular social group or political opinion, is outside the country of his nationality and is unable or owing to such fear, is unwilling to avail himself of the protection of that country."

Leaving everything behind for an unknown future and facing drastic and life-changing risks, at one's own person and as witness leaves behind a large number of people the urgently need help to recover and heal. While escaping war zones, hunger and injustice, they delivered themselves to risky journeys in the hope of a better future, only to find themselves struggling to survive in tiny boats, often sexually harassed, robbed and kept in detention camps for months.

The few that arrived in a safe place with available psycho-physiological care, financial means for survival, shelter and trauma therapy shed a different light on previous trauma studies. Why am I writing this? Isn't it common sense? Does not everybody know this?

I think everybody knows but as soon as photos of overcrowded camps appear on the news a dehumanisation happens in the eyes of the spectator and once the refugees arrived in our countries, the government and the people expect nothing else from them but to either leave to their home countries or visually disappear in some integration—called loss of identity. I still dream of an integration that allows diversity, cultural independence and social security, tolerance and connection in order to heal from Traumatic events that most of us cannot even think of without having nightmares.

The traumatic background in the cases of most refugees is multiple and complex, including at least between three and five traumatising incidents that happened to each individual, such as:

- loss of home
- loss of social status
- loss of financial background
- loss of family member(s), friend(s)
- loss of cultural context
- sexual assault
- violence
- language barriers
- insecurity about the coming years, visa status
- injuries
- threatened by guns, knives, explosives

- life-threatening experiences or observing someone in a life-threatening situation
- illness
- depression

Unaccompanied children often face even more traumatising situations. Loneliness, loss of cultural identity and the lack of family support leave them vulnerable for life when no help is given as a preventative to overcome their isolation.

Survivors of Sudden and Massive Impacts and PTSD

However, in Europe, the group of traumatised patients due to gun violence, mass shootings remain an exception, at least for now. While school children in the US often suffer from being exposed gun violence in schools and colleges or deeply fear such, extreme mass terror events are rare in Europe. The recovery rate from PTS of survivors is relatively high due to quick help and often provided compensation by the government(in Europe).

However, survivors are often suffering from prolonged symptoms if no professional help is at hand or the process of recognition is as a victim is difficult, unclear, devaluating or even doubting the victim's experience.

Some of my patients are survivors of terror attacks, like the Bataclan attack in Paris (2015), the Christmas market in Berlin (2016) or other unpredictable, rare, brutal events, such as knife attacks or gun violence. A significant influence on my work and my view on such events in the sense of the importance of proper after care as well as meaning making solutions was made by Kapil, who survived the 4-day terror attacks in Mumbai in the Taj Hotel, 2008.

Traumatised Helpers and First Aid Responders

A number of patients were doctors of emergency rooms or helpers like first aid responders, helpers in refugee camps, being out on boats in the Mediterranean or South China Sea to rescue people, they are fireman, police or nurses.

Their situation is so different in many ways of other victims as they are hardly recognised as being constantly exposed. Many of those first responders are experiencing the effects of their constant exposure only after decades of work. Their increasing experience of physical discomfort, nervousness, depression, irritability, lack of energy, problematic relationships, feeling of loneliness, sleeplessness and so on have been downplayed or even hidden from friends and family so often a diagnose of PTSD comes late.

The inability to share the experience with people who are close creates a distance. A void in life that only be compensated by relieving the stress again and again in the need to act out. It is important to Many traumatised patients treated by me and my assistants at the Society of Friends of first-aid helpers as well as long-term helpers; they experienced trauma by having daily encounters with the toxicity of the images and stories of broken life stories, injured bodies and desperation.

Yet again, even similar to the experience of the soldiers, the first aid responder has a high standard in society and will most likely receive quick aid and financial compensation. These factors increase their options for recovery.

Why The basic of study on trauma in soldiers might not hit the majority of traumatised civilians and others

The recent research on trauma and PTSD done in the homogenous group of traumatised US soldiers and those with PTSD might not be relevant for a more diverse group. Their traumatic incidents mostly resemble each other, as they are the most common ones during the war:

-   combat injuries
-   combat observing trauma
-   loss of comrades
-   actively killing soldiers
-   actively killing civilians
-   the conflict between religious and social meanings and order

Suppose research on a group with quite defined outlines represents all other individuals who do not match the above criteria. It is necessary to understand the differences in developing trauma to design a fitting therapy concept for the victim. War has justified murder, rape and any violence to save the nation, confusing right or wrong.

43

Rape is always wrong. One should even consider rape not as a sexual assault but as violent crime. Making the shit in definition from sex to crime will put the victim into a very different light. (F. J., private conversation 20.10.2020)

Recent Research on Co-Morbidity
The Relationship Between Psychological Trauma and Substance Abuse

The publications of Dr Gabor Mate. Gabor Mate is a Hungarian-Canadian physician residing in Toronto, Canada. Originating from a Hungarian Jewish Holocaust survivor's family, he analysed his previous addictive behaviour. His work on addiction is ground-breaking as he adds an important change to the viewpoint of the addict. His question is not: *What do you lose by being an addict, but what do you gain from it.* (Mate, 2013*)*

In this change of perspective, he tries to find the key to treating the addict by understanding the pain and the void. His focus was not on what, when or how the trauma occurred, but how survivors adapted to their survival.

His understanding of addiction does not base on merely neuroscience, but on empathy.

Mate: *Addiction is manifested in any behaviour that a person craves, finds temporary relief or pleasure in but suffers the negative consequences as a result of and yet has difficulty giving up. In brief: craving, relief, pleasure, suffering, impaired control. Note that this definition is not restricted to drugs but could encompass almost any human behaviour, from sex to eating to shopping to gambling to extreme sports to tv to compulsive internet use: the list is endless.*

"I am not going to ask you what you were addicted to", I often say to people, "nor when, nor for how long. Only, whatever your addictive focus, what did it offer to you? What did you like about it? What, in the short term did it give you that you liked so much?"

And universally, the answers are: It helped me escape emotional pain— helped me deal with stress—gave me peace of mind—a sense of connection with others—a sense of control. (Mate, transcript, TED Talk, The power of addiction, the addiction to power, 2013)

His experience in Toronto's sad and lonely suburbs, working as a physician mainly with drug addicts, comes to the conclusion about the onset of trauma and how people deal with the pain and the void. His focus is on the person and their way of adapting to pain, not his view on drugs. He believes addiction is not separate from trauma. However, not all trauma survivors develop addictive behaviour, but any addictive behaviour is rooted in childhood trauma.

However, the treatment in the case of co-morbidity is problematic. Prioritising is important as co morbidity can have fatal results if unknown, there could be self-harm or harming others, organ failure and other light to severe physical problems alone, not to mention the psychological impact of withdrawal. All the pain that has been suppressed with substances lashes back. The trauma as a root of substance abuse explains why most withdrawals without significant therapy on the traumatic history will not be successful and relapse occurs.

Bessel Van der Kolk, Peter Levine

Peter Levine became popular with his books on Trauma published for a wider audience and even self-help guide books. Books such as "In An Unspoken Voice: How the body releases trauma and restores goodness" (2010), "Waking the tiger, healing trauma" (1997), "Trauma and memory, brain and body in a search for the living past: A practical guide for understanding and working with traumatic memory" (2015) were written for psychotherapists but as well as for interested non-medical practitioners and even for traumatised people themselves.

His publications include several self-practice chapters for the traumatised patient with a simple, optimistic outlook on healing oneself through exercises. Bessel van der Kolk, often working with Levine, has published books and articles for social workers, psychological or psychiatric therapists, less to the public.

Patients in case studies presented by Bessel van der Kolk and P. Levine (both working in the field for almost 40 years) show depression and substance use disorder (SUD), polysubstance abuse (recreational drugs in combination with alcohol and prescribed medication) and have conducted more than one sign of disorder in their life after the traumatic event, in line with Minkoff's appeal that medical professionals must recognise that comorbidity is not the exception but the norm.

Unlike Gabor Mate, with whom Bessel van der Kolk and Peter Levine are closely associated, they focus on emotional, physical experiences. They all have in common, not the incident itself should repeat over and over again in therapy to integrate it in the personal narrative, but that all life *after* trauma needs understanding and support. Peter Levine and Bessel van der Kolk agree on a somatic experience through trauma and start healing from psycho-emotional bodywork.

In some techniques they propose, the ancient Indian origin of their practices is seen. An example is a famously recorded session from Peter Levine with a veteran. The veteran is asked to hum:

"MMMMMMMH," allowing him to control his distressed arousal. Their focus on breath work, drama and even expressive dance is displaying traditional healing methods in a standardised form for merely the predominantly western patient.

Another influential voice in trauma therapy is the German psychiatrist Michaela Huber. She stresses certain aspects of the client/therapist relationship.

Different from psychoanalysis, she suggests empathic behaviour towards the patient. Her belief is that this approach does not trigger a victim/aggressor relationship memory. The role of the therapist should change and develop during treatment. She draws a clear line between trauma therapy, psychoanalysis and "explanation-interpretation."

For example: "What You mean is—" she states that this is more or less a typical traumatising situation in which the aggressor creates the "real" meaning of the situation. In cases of sexual harassment: "I know you want it as well," "You said no, but I know that you meant yes."

A key phrase of the conversation on her therapeutic approach is, the patient asking: "What do you think I should do now?" and the therapist answers, "What do *You* think what you should do now?"

Different from Bessel van der Kolk and the above therapists, she counts on intellectual understanding and relationship-based experiences during therapy. Experience-based relationship mean the safe relationship of patient/therapist to safely re-experience the trauma the trauma and develop the relationship during treatment as a model. She uses pictures and narratives. Her main request is to stay abstinent beside the empathy and not provide any shelter, touch, intimacy, personal engagement or other help to the patient. Researchers differ in their understanding of the behaviour of traumatised patients.

Like Michaela Huber, König sees it as the consequence of the trauma, while others, like Mate and Levine, believe it is an adaptation to the trauma. Research papers and publications seem to be like the description of an elephant by a group of blind people: it is round when touching the legs, soft and smooth when touching the husk, windy and floppy when touching the husked ear. For complex disturbances, trauma alone cannot define clearly and coherently by one single term alone. It is too complicated and too much of an individual experience, depending on:

- age,
- sex,
- time,
- repetition,
- location,
- resilience,
- follow up safety,
- family and
- other diversities of the experience.

Gabor Mate states that we have to understand why some people recover fully and, even in a short period of time, whilst other seem not to recover at all—signs like stable relationships can be promising as signs of full recovery, of a successful integration of the trauma in the victim's life—even as a learning tool. That obviously can add meaning to life (here is coming into play, from a different point of view).

However, in the same empathetic tenor, what I feel is the key to understand the depths of ayurvedic treatments: they provide meaning in life by restoring the ability to connect—and he continues. He says that others cannot recover as they lost any meaning in life and their social life has become unbearable so that chronic pain, disease and addictions are the marks on a road to an early death.

Understanding the complexity and diversity of defining trauma and developing treatment plans on the concept of memory is crucial. Neuroscience is becoming the guide into the dark realms.

Understanding what, how and where memory is stored helps memories fade under circumstances and conditions. In Neuroscience we are still learning how memory can affect our whole system.

Beginning from thinking and experiencing the world as a safe or unsafe place from a single event and moment onwards:

- How does memory influence our capacity to enjoy happiness or remain in fear and depression?
- How can memory affect our cognitive abilities?
- How does memory affect our ability to build strong and healthy relationships or even reproduce the distress-loaded experiences repeatedly?
- How our memory influences all biochemical aspects of our physical being?

Research is therefore entering the trauma discussion from two ends these days:

- understanding memory
- understanding response

The goal would be to alter the memory and, finally, the distress response. Julia Shaw, a behavioural and neuro—scientist who works as a professor as well as a profiler for the police, states that memories of trauma are highly emotional.

Julia Shaw, 2016. She states that our memory of emotional events is flawed. As a scientist and not a therapist, she criticises therapeutic approaches based on memory contents. She criticises Freud for his assumption that we do have an unconscious mind. An assumption that has become so common that even every child has heard about.

However, we should take in consideration what Freud's methods were to claim the revolutionary findings this is where Julia Shaw is breaking into the taboo of western psychologist thinking—Freud was convinced that there is an unconscious mind that stores unwanted and unpleasant memories and gets therefore actively suppressed by the conscious mind, including unwanted desires.

She continues in her book that Freud stated all-female trauma dates back to childhood abuse and if a patient denies such an event, he automatically takes this from there as a proof because she is in denial. I find her work extremely important as she sheds a light on the concrete building of western therapy.

Freud, as she says, came to the conclusion that all of this could be treated in therapy by the use of imaginary reproduction. Despite protests that sexual abuse had not occurred, Freud insisted on his theory by proving the women wrong because of their denial.

We can clearly see that there are many different scientific and psychological interpretations and approaches toward the mechanisms and content of memory. Shaw argues that there is also a potential downside to therapeutic strategies based on recalling and verbalising the traumatic events, particularly in group therapy, where patients are overwhelmed with traumatic stories.as Shaw's main study topic is memory and how memory can easily be altered, her work is groundbreaking for all therapies that are based on recalling the (maybe) memory.

The more often patients talk about their trauma, the faster their brain reproduces the (painful) memory. Each time patients recall the trauma, it reinforces and automatises, adding new memories.

We should not forget that therapists, like Freud, might also create false contents. French, another researcher on false memory, extends Shaw's opinion that there is no evidence for this psycho-analytic dogma of repressed memories, instead, he says, psychotherapy itself can be a ground to create false memory just by its setting.

Patient **A** who was attending a group therapy session in a psycho-somatic hospital, told me: "They are all so depressed, it depresses me even more."

Another example can be patient **U,** who initially did not recall too many detailed memories of the terrorist attack at the Christmas Market in Berlin. She had to quickly stop group therapy because she felt that the memories of other participants displayed so much graphic violence and triggered her previous traumatic memories. Now, she states she has a better memory of the event formed through other people's narratives: "There are these horrible pictures I cannot get out of my head."

Trauma therapy is not an easy task. It requires experience and stamina and knowledge to detect the subtle information, to withstand the sometimes upcoming impatience, to remain empathetic, to withstand seduction and keep an overview.

When there are contradicting concepts in western psychology, psychiatry and neuroscience which then point into different directions such as pharmaceuticals, behavioural, confrontational, analytic, EMDR, shamanic, hypnotherapeutic or any other treatment it seems that it is up to the patient to fit in these models not that the models can be adapted to the patient. This is my main criticism of western models and what I see as the greatest advantage of Ayurveda therapy, including trauma and PTSD.

The patients cannot be standardised or better, customised to the options of treatments. The varieties of the patients' educational, social, gender, sex, family, heritage, upbringing, cultural backgrounds differ as much as the varieties and number of traumatising events are countless. There are multiple causes and infinite options for the experience of traumatic psychological impact. Some patients survive multiple traumas without showing any significant changes in their behaviour and meaning-making, different to those who develop addiction and symptoms of constant distress after a "minor" impact.

In some cases, some even started to live a better, happier and more meaningful life following a traumatic experience. Some victims reproduce their trauma in their daily lives and relationships, some pass it on to the next generation and some become self-aware, self-reflecting and caring. Some patients, however, lose all sense of self-worth and some suddenly think of themselves as goddesses.

As a trauma therapist (which I would actually deny to be one as I am treating in a holistic concept), I believe one of the most perplexing aspects of trauma is the enormous difference between those patients who show or do not show signs of aftershock and those who remember or do not remember the incident. However, the ones that suffer need adequate help quickly.

The standard view and concept is that the Trauma experiences and aftermaths like PTSD are solely psychological problems. This does not take physiological changes and distress in account that have an imprint on our health care system in the sense of: An increased number of heart problems and heart attacks in trauma patients, high blood pressure, under/overeating, sleeplessness, addiction that patients seek help at their General Practitioner and get on the journey to meet their psychotherapist.

Understanding the body-mind continuum is rare and holistic therapies are generally not scientific. However, Diabetes, cancer, Multiple Sclerosis and AMLS seem to be related to severe distress as Gabor Mate writes in his book: *When the body says No, Exploring the Stress-Disease Connection.* He states that there is a possible relationship between stress, impaired immunity and illness.

He uses the term "the concept of diseases of adaption", a phrase of Hans Seyle's. he continues that the fight and flight response is there for what it ever was helpful: escaping and surviving stressful experiences. However, these days, the constant stressors for most people are emotional. So we find ourselves in lifestyles or emotions that are destroying ourselves.

The variety of methods on how to treat the victims of trauma is vast and uncountable. Treatment within the general health insurance system in Germany leads to separation of symptoms as all medical personal is specialised and not holistic. Receiving psychotherapy, therefore, could be paid for, but it is usually a long way and often needs extra surveillance a limited number of hours can lead to.

Disappointment, a feeling of neglect, helplessness and even suicide when further help is rejected. A common answer to patients/therapists requests to a prolonged treatment allowance is: if there was no improvement in the sense of diminishing the symptoms there is no healing expected, therefore the payment stops. The common psychotherapist is often not experienced enough and their education has not equipped them for trauma therapy.

Some trauma patients received devaluating or irritating statements from their therapist, for instance: Anh (name changed) is a survivor of the boat people of South Vietnam in the late 90ies. After she had reported her therapist about her feelings of weakness, fear, an increase in heartbeat and sleeplessness, she was told to "get your act together."

Other patients had been exposed to judgmental comments before. Their therapists could not find anything wrong with their past. Throughout the beginning of the therapy sessions, the patients could not reveal their trauma content easily because of shame, fear, dissociation, memory problems, young age or other.

Some did not have access to their traumatising history. Patients might have even felt at a dead end on the road after the trauma diagnosis. Being a trauma patient might jeopardise their personal life and career and might not even help the recovery in the future as there is a stigma; the patients have a "mental disorder, they are mad".

Most private insurances in Germany, for example, have strict regulations not accepting patients with previous psychiatric diagnoses. Furthermore, many German health insurance providers do not reimburse complementary medicine and complementary healing offers such as Ayurveda, Yoga Therapy, Acupuncture or herbalism.

Listening to patients who had reached out desperately to find justice, help, support or compensation brings a flashlight into a dysfunctional health system.

Some patients had to go back to full-time work while dealing with a history of rape, severe physical damage and emotional devastation. If this is not possible because their PTSD symptoms are too damaging, they often will not receive further government support and end up poor and devastated.

The waiting list for PTSD therapy is long. In Berlin, Germany, alone the waiting time for patients even with acute significant self-harming behaviour and acute suicidal attempt ranges from months to years. Most of the patients have been treated symptomatically by their physicians with anti-depressants, painkillers or sleepers. A vicious circle begins. Medical treatments mostly leave the patients unsatisfied as the symptoms persist. Meanwhile, addiction to substances can arise and lead to more attempts of adapting to their illness instead of healing.

The Ayurveda Approach: Ancient Empiric Wisdom of the Universal Relationship of Man and Nature in the Context of Trauma

In Ayurveda, we are aiming to generate a holistic view of the patient in order to provide a holistic treatment. However, the differentiation in diagnostic terms as what is called *trauma* is difficult in the complex socio-philosophical-medical context of Ayurveda.

Eastern medical concepts, such as Ayurveda, Tibetan or other Oriental Medicine systems like Chinese, Korean, Japanese traditional medicine, are based on empirical research and philosophical approaches towards life, death, health, happiness and the function of the mind itself. Eastern medicine permanently embeds a holistic concept, unlike western biomedicine matters and facts where philosophy is not a crucial part of scientific research.

In eastern traditions, the individual well-being cannot be separated from the well-being of the family, community or land/country. Environmental issues are as important as emotional or physical disturbances and recovery. The world and every being are in a networking context, where a change disrupts all other systems. A comparison, therefore, is difficult, if not impossible, as western biomedical views are analytical, which means that they are breaking down a whole picture into minor parts (blood results, cell cultures, etc.).

At the same time, traditional Eastern Medicine has an inductive-synthetic approach (Manfred Porkert, 1996), meaning integrating as many aspects as possible into the picture and observing the connections of every part as a representation of the whole. Therefore, Eastern Medicine is considered not as an individualistic healing system but a holistic one in the whole overall embracing and connecting sense of the word "holistic".

Any traditional medicine system, western traditional Medicine and Alternative Medicine, Indigenous medicines of different kinds, shamans they all have their own rules and assumptions based on empirical wisdom and experiences, close observation and accepting results from the philosophical framework.

However, to understand the specialties fundamental differences in diagnosis and treatment, it is necessary to have a close view ayurvedic and yoga medical and philosophical terms and meanings. Empirical research has been generated and collected over hundreds or thousands of years, including immeasurable case studies displaying success and failure. Empirical knowledge is not ideological. It serves nothing more than the interest of the patient. If a system is inefficient over time, it's most likely to disappear.

Ayurveda and yoga display collections of wisdom and philosophy spanning several millennia. The effectiveness of ancient systems of knowledge and practice, such as Ayurveda and Yoga, is evident in their continued existence. Nowadays, modern laboratory tests can verify claimed healing properties of herbal medicine or other medical interventions.

An international research source for such tests is *PubMed*, the official American research platform that hosts a specific Ayurveda section. India, represented in AYUSH, also keeps several research platforms that deal with analysing laboratory research data. Whether the isolation of substances can genuinely reflect the holistic mindset and concept of medical intervention is the question; however, these studies are helpful to contribute to a critical review of ancient plant medicine and its risks and benefits.

The western mind must undergo the challenge to rethink the body-mind relation to understand the inner core of ayurvedic or yoga wisdom. In the tradition of Samkhya philosophy, there is no separation of body and mind. The Cartesian influence has divided the living being into two entities and we even have to use two words in order to describe that there are not two entities but only one single continuum.

Ayurveda and yoga state a continuum of interrelation, density and subtleness, from the finest aspects of the being to the largest. Still, there are no two separate sections, as if they could ever exist separately. However, Prof. Ram

Manohar states there is a concept of psychiatry in Ayurveda that comes into play once the emotional factors of the person are shattered. (Ram Manohar, 2018)

In the sciences and concepts of yoga and ayurveda, the function of the mind and body continuum reveals clear terms and practical guidance. Empirical knowledge and hundreds of techniques for self-inquiry are laid out.

Starting from social and metaphysical thinking in yoga, through the *yamas* and *niyamas* (how to react responsible towards oneself and the community), to physical exercise in yoga (*asana*), deep meditation (*dhyana*) and finally liberation (*samadhi*). From breathing inquiry (*pranayama*) to the daily routine (*dinarcharya*), detailed descriptions of practice, cause and effect are structured and explained. *Ahara/vihara* (nutrition and lifestyle) are pillars of rules, ethics and philosophical outlines.

The often-used meaning of the word *yoga* is vaguely translated into "unity, connection." Ayurveda usually translates as the science of life and death.

Historical influences have not been able to erase the richness of philosophies from India. In fact, every new episode in the history of the enormous subcontinent has added to the richness of beliefs, customs and manners. Until today, India provides a spectrum of ideas and philosophies as an experience of diversity. These experiences are joined together into one bigger and multi-diverse picture.

This picture reflects and incorporates the multiple societal changes through invaders, natural disasters and golden ages within a historical timeline from the ancient past to the present day. It accepts and integrates traditions from the highest university standards with lab tests to procedures summarised under the name of shamanism.

From *rasaushadhis* (refining toxic substances to lose their toxicity) to recite mantras. From touch and massage therapy to sexual therapy and child wish (*vajrkarana*). Ayurveda and yoga can renounce the world or indulge fully but consciously in all its temptations in India's medical tradition. Indian philosophies allow everything to integrate into the picture of life and meaning.

It spans from the high altitude of the Himalayas of Jammu and Kashmir, influencing other Oriental traditions, like Tibetan, Mongolian and Chinese Traditional Medicine, down to the damp swamps or deep jungles of Kerala and Karnataka. It covers knowledge of medical plants and traditions from the vast deserts of Rajasthan and those from agricultural settlements.

It integrates cow-based medicine of Uttar Pradesh to coconut oil preparations from Sri Lanka. It covers most uncountable medical traditions in a subcontinent home to almost 1,500 official languages and about the same number of so-called minor languages and dialects. Most medical traditions are passed down from generations of *vaidyas (ayurvedic doctors)* to their offspring or students. ayurvedic universities date even 3,000 years back (Encyclopaedia Britannica, 2019).

They often hosted hundreds of scholars even then. A devastating interruption of knowledge happened when British colonialists forbade all ayurvedic medical practices, closed universities and forced India to retreat from its rich traditions. Translating Sanskrit or Arabic medical terms into English language and thinking therefore has confused concepts and meanings during this period and up until now.

The Concept of Samkhya

Samkhya philosophy is the most widely used concept in ayurveda and classical yoga. *Samkhya* is only one of the hundreds of concepts in Indian philosophies. The embedment of Ayurveda as several different yoga schools conceptualise their primary explanations from the creation of the universe to the formation of matter (*mahabhutas*, often translated as "elements" because of their prominent solid figures).

The system of *Samkhya* describes subtle energies from emotional aspects of consciousness to immense elements. The substantial delicate parts are the *gunas*, namely *sattva, rajas and tamas.*

The *gunas* and the *doshas* are primary qualities for disease prevention, treatment, a holistic view of the patient and their relation to nature and the life cycle.

The Gunas:

- *Sattva* is a passive, tranquil state. It is stable, not as much as *tamas*, but stable enough to be flexible and adapt to maintain equilibrium.
- *Tamas* is elsewhere often translated in western texts as "passive" in the sense of lazy, dull, uninspired, which might be a cultural misunderstanding.

In western culture, quick changes and individualism are preferred ideological parameters. Other translations are adhesive, gluey, connecting, heavy. *Tamas* is the most inert aspect of the universe. Inertia also means stability and connectivity as well. D. Frawley translates *tamas* even as a principle considered like love as it is passive, stable, connecting and maintaining.

- *Rajas* is an embodiment of dominance, guidance and direction. It is the warrior aspect, the drive, the willpower. It is the sperm penetrating the ovum, the seed. It is often a favoured state of mind in the west.

The Three Doshas Concerning the Human Body and Their Actions

The *doshas* are a complex system of understanding the world of matter and beyond. They are described as material as well as momentum in time and space. Although this system is simplifying and unscientific in the west, it reflects a highly refined approach to understanding action, the reaction inside the body and interrelated action and response with the world and the person. The world, as such, includes all living beings and describes the seasons and emotional-physiological appearance and modifications of interrelations of every human being.

Shiv Sharma describes the *doshas* as a physical-physiological-psychological-organic complex of phenomena. (Prof. M. Mittwede, 1998).

The above terminology reflects the multi-dividing pattern of western scientific thinking through the descriptive analogy. While Ayurveda represents the idea of a holistic treatment, the practitioner has to live and understand the holistic approaches. western scientists, in contrast, have to separate actions, forms, matter, levels, mind and body.

Prof. Martin Mittwede writes in "Der Ayurveda", that *so* many trials of interpretation are existing, shows that the doshas are something that is not so easy to grasp and obviously like other senses data. He senses that the forwarded explanations of the doshas seem to be often more likely an expression of the scientific background of the author opposed to an explicit analysis of what the ayurvedic classics actually intended with the terms dosha, vata, pitta, kapha.

Vata, pitta and *kapha* are composed of the five basic natural qualities, often translated as "element" (Sanskrit: *Mahabhutas.)* They display basic qualities associated with their natural attributes:

The *mahabhutas* or primary substances are:

Prithvi (earth)

Apah/Jala (water)

Agni/Tejas (fire)

Vayu (air, wind)

Akasha (space, ether)

The *Mahabhutas* appear in paired combinations as *doshas*:

Prthvi (earth) and *jala* (water) are the elementary forms/functions of *kapha dosha.*

Jala (water) and *agni* (fire) are the elementary forms/functions for *pitta dosha.*

Vayu (air) and *akasha* (space) are the elementary forms/functions for *vata dosha.*

The *Mahabhutas* form, shape and qualify the *doshas*. So that *vayu* and *akasha* are the elements that create *vata dosha, jala* and *tejas* create the *pitta dosha* and *prithvi* and *jala* create *kapha dosha*. The *doshas* are a person's constitution, an object, a plant, a medicine.

Elements of Three Doshas

Vata	*Pitta*	*Kapha*
dry	oily	heavy
light	sharp	slow
cold	(penetrating)	cold
rough	hot	oily
subtle	light	slimy (smooth)
mobile	mobile	dense
clear	liquid	soft
		static (stable)
		cloudy (sticky)

"The activity that can be observed is dual: in harmonious or disturbed pattern."

(Prof. Martin Mittwede,1998)

Simplifying the concepts might allow a quicker overview of the ideas of the *doshas*. Simplifying, however, bears risks. It might give the impression of parascientific expertise, even pseudo-science, which the recent Wikipedia remarks from a wrong quotation of Prof. Ram Manohar explained.

The body chart allows a quick overview of the *doshas'* concepts and terms, relations and interrelations. It displays a structure of judgement and observation. However, this structure might vary from author to author. Each author directs the focus on their research according to their preferences.

It is important to understand that the following table refers to a healthy state of the *doshas* and a balanced state. Yet, it allows a simple understanding of the concepts in the ayurvedic context.

	VATA	*PITTA*	*KAPHA*
BODY FRAME	Lean to thin, irregular, short or very tall, long extremities, knuckles visible (the marathon runner)	proportionate, athletic in healthy condition (the iron man)	Round body frame, broad, evenly proportioned the weight lifter
WEIGHT and FEATURES relating form and shape	hard to gain, little fat, lose skin, hyper-elastic skin, stretchmarks, hair growth on breasts, ovary region, abdominal, back of the spine, cold hands	Stable, gains muscles with ease Warm body, soft warm feeling, warm hands, warm feet	Gains weight easily, hard to lose fat, cold hands, damp hands and feet
SKINTYPES	dark powdered and thin, shine through with blue arteries and veins showing, often dark spots or darker skin patches (under the eyes, around the wrists), choppy, dry	warm, light and reddish, (English rose) slightly orangy colour, shiny, radiant look. In case of Pitta aggravation red puffy upper body and face	cool, fair and oily, (comment by the author: *kapha* does not tan easily but stays somewhat whitish in complexion
HAIR	dry, thin, skin patches	straight, fine, early balding or white	Oily texture, curly, thick, wavy
EYES	Gray, blue or unusual colour, bi colour	Brown, green, hazel, light brown,	blue, dark brown, big, sensual, light

59

NAILS	dry, ridged, instable, fine, breaking easily, fine, small	clear, well-formed, pliable, strong	square, white, even, strong and oily
APPETITE	Irregular, easy to skip a meal, loses appetite under stress	Intense, getting irritable with no food, under stress overeating	Consistent appetite, even under stress
STOOL	constipated, irregular, small quantity like sheep portions, gas, bloated	loose, regular, large quantity, formed	slow, steady, moderate quantity, oily, formed
SWEAT	Hardly, mostly fishy smell, close to the body, sweat patches on the lower back, cold sweat	Profuse, smell of leather or acid smell in sickness, big sweat patches under the arms, on the upper back	Easy sweating, in healthy state odourless or smell of fruit, in sickness: apple smell, sticky
STAMINA	Shifting, quickly exhausted, longer recovery rate	moderate, driven with competition, easily recovered, over doing	excellent, endurant, easily recovered if healthy, depressed and lazy in sickness
Sleep Pattern	Variable, late bedtime, waking up at night, light sleep	moderate, sound, in sickness: difficult falling asleep due to late eating, over working or using alcohol in the evening to unwind	long, deep, wakes up refreshed, in sickness: oversleepin g, too many hours sleeping, feeling drowsy or hang over

60

Doshas: Emotional Characteristics

RELATION TO THE WORLD	fearful, indecisive, nervous, perceptive constantly changing and trying to adapt or try something new. unsteady	intelligent, arrogant, successful strong opinions leadership narcissistic traits self-righteousne ss in sickness, healthy moral if balanced	calm, stable, stubborn tendency to lazy ness, over waiting before decision making, little drive to change situations
MEMORY	learns quickly, lack of concentrati on on one subject forgets quickly remember details but not the whole	learns quickly and has a good memory for broader content forgets slowly	learns slowly, forgets slowly
SPEECH	erratic, talkative	decisive, articulate	slow, cautious
SPIRITUALI TY	spiritually, disciplined	tendency to material success	fundament al, material
Dreamy times	Dreaming of flying white objects, of the sky but also of fearful, situations, wakes up from dreams erratic	violent, intense	watery, sensual, long sequences
SEXlife	Easily started but losing interest quickly, variable, not	hot, intense, easy to perform. Tendency to affairs because of	warm, enduring, loves touch and comfort.

	consistent in relationshi p as needs a lot of time alone. Needs comfort but dislikes touch	intense sexual desire	

Our body type chart seems to be more superficial than it actually is. One needs time to get into the skill of observing in the context of Ayurveda. One needs to be enabled to understand that prakriti is the original self—structure that represents karmic as well often related to genetic dominance. As genetics need a factor to get into action, so are the Mahabhutas and, finally, the doshas emerge. But even the quality of the doshas, often translated as error, can only be a factor of Unmada, disease or other ailments, if the conditions are there that create a dominance.

The dominance of doshas are easily mistaken in the west to disqualify individuals and also to insist that there is a determination. It is not. It is a constant movement that only can maintain a healthy balance if it is not blocked or exaggerated, but flowing freely.

The *doshas* are the basic concept in Ayurveda for explaining health and disease and finding ways to maintain or restore balance. The *doshas* explicitly define a holistic point of view with an individualistic approach towards health and sickness. The uniqueness of each being is not a contradiction to the unity of all existence.

The activities of the *doshas* are governed by twenty *gunas* (not including *gunas sattva, rajas and tamas)* and or qualities. These qualities are opposite pairs like hard, soft, cold, hot, rough, smooth, soft, etc. The three *doshas: vata, pitta and kapha,* substantially incorporate all information about the unfolding of existence.

In yoga practice, the longing for the reunion of two primordial forces, *purusha*, as the individualised aspect of the original soul and *prakriti,* the primordial matter, reduce all the activity (karma) to find the purity and stillness before any creation took place (*sattva, samadhi*). The dualistic explanations in *Samkhya* transcend the duality of life and death, mind and matter to dissolve in until moksha or samadhi end the cycle of creation (*samsara*).

An Inquiry Into Medical Terms and Understandings in Different Cultures: *Ama*

Ama is a profound concept in Ayurveda that can perfectly illustrate the problems of translation, interpretation and cultural misuse of concepts. *Ama* is a harmful substance that slows down processes and causes disturbance and illness. *Ama* is a crucial word in Ayurvedic Medicine. *Ama* could be interpreted as "undigested, raw" but must not translate as "detox". If the agni or digestive fire is not strong enough or the person's food and lifestyle choice are not congruent with the ability, we see the development of ama.

Amamannarasamkechitkedittumalasanchyam
Prathma dosa dushti cha kechit amam pracakshate.

Unfortunately, *ama* removal is often wrongly translated as DETOX in the west, often even used synonym by Ayurveda practitioners. In western concepts of impurity eradication named DETOX in natural medicine, it is very unspecific, both in what and how it is removed. Mostly laxative teas or enemas are considered a "detox" method for ailments that do not necessarily include *ama's* vast concept. Detox stands for improving physical and mental performance, cleanliness, purity.

In particular, so-called liver cleanses contribute to a large number of non-alcoholic fatty liver cases in the US and Europe. Professor Ram Manohar from Amrita College, Kollam Kerala highlighted at the International Ayurveda Conference in Nadiad/Gujarat in 2018,that if we use the word "Detox", we then have to prove what we are talking about. We have to prove that we eliminate substances and what substances.

In classic Ayurveda, *ama* is a complex concept with precisely described measures on how to detect it and how to eliminate it:

Ushmano 'lpa balatvena dhatum adyama pachitam
Dushtam amashaya gatam rasam amam prachashate.

Meaning, if the first dhatu is affected by impairment of the digestive fire, it starts the process of ama. Ama can also be formed by unprocessed emotions, like unexpressed anger, fear, greed, envy, shame and even too much elation which leads to mental ama. As ama is sticky, it diminishes the digestive fire even more.

Speaking about the gunas, the mental activity is clouded and we observe the stickiness be the person's thoughts stuck in the past. A good agni, a good clear digestion on all levels of perception, allows us to be in the moment and observe the past but not be stuck in the past. It is an integrating process on all levels of the being. A good agni allows clarity to penetrate and purify all dhatus, srotas and other structures of the body as well the as the mental activities. Being in the present moment is the way to heal.

Charaka describes *Ama* based on its symptoms, not the way of its removal:

- stiffness or heaviness in the body/mind
- lack of inspiration
- feeling of being unwell, numbed, shattered
- lack of appetite, digestive disorder
- sluggish digestion. blocked digestion, bloated abdomen
- sinking stool, stinking body and excrement odour
- thick coating of the tongue
- sticky phlegm discharge
- lack of clarity of mind and senses

It is important to leave the western Cartesian concept of a duality of mind and matter behind to understand the differences of western thinking. One must observe the deep complexity of a philosophical system that instead describes existence as a continuum of unfolding and connection (significantly different to think of two pieces—mind and body and then nothing. Life and death are not separated. Whatever we try to put into action is wrong from our points of view, cannot overcome duality thinking, so imprinted, tricking us).

Ayurveda looks at the unfolding of life as being in a constant movement of creation and decays with individualised self-care according to the *doshas* and *gunas*, understanding the cycles of daily life and aging.

Ayurvedic practices care for maintaining health and providing a cure for illnesses. Yoga focuses on understanding our existence's mental and psychological features through self-inspection. Self-inquiry and self-care/cure introduce the two sciences deriving from the same source of *Samkhya*.

However, their ways and goals are different. In functional appliances for the patient, they join with treatment plans. Yoga and Ayurveda create a stable system of self-reflection, self-responsibility, meaning-making and an understanding of achieving inner stability and taking care of one's health, family, the community, the country and the environment.

Translation of Clinical Sanskrit Terms

As Sanskrit is a very complex language and translation depend on the context and the sentence, meaning and the speaker, it is almost impossible to translate the meaning into any other language without interpreting the texts. Interpretation means the words adapt to the different culture's meanings. The original Sanskrit terms are kept in this book as much as possible to avoid misunderstandings.

Sanskrit is a language that inquires philosophical questions and teaches understanding of the mysterious, the infinite, the connection and even daily topics. It is a language of medicine and can be used in households; it is the oldest language with writing that looks back into a history of thousands of years till our times. It is spoken today rarely and then mostly only in Brahmin families. Sanskrit is not part of the cultural heritage of India's Muslim community and is only used by Hindu families.

Details of the 8 psychological factors and behavioural factors used in Ayurveda studies on mental health. Manas refers to the thought, affect and emotional aspect of the mind. Therefore, delusions and delusional ideas and states of mind and emotions like, depression, overall uncontained excitement, elation, anxiety etc. are assessed under this factor.

Buddhi (ya buddhi nishcayatnika Ca. Sa 1/33) represents the instance of the intellect, the clear decision making and problem-solving aspects. *Sanjna jnana* represents awareness of surroundings, connection and response to stimuli and allows orientation. Responsiveness and attention only can arise and create parts of consciousness.

Smriti allows memory. memory is a complex process, starting from short term to long term. Memory is not a simple imprint of what has been seen, heard, observed in the past but in fact a narrowing of past experiences. Memory can be easily falsified or changed due to emotional impact. Bhakti is the quality that allows us to feel devotion, surrender. It is adaption but not in a negative way like the adaption to trauma, but in a blissful, joyful devotional state.

However, more mundane aspects of bhakti are the joy of good food, finding pleasure in hobbies, study, work and, in general, in all beneficial activities. Experiencing and sharing sexual pleasure is a quality that arises from <u>bhakti</u>. Habits and temperament that are expressed in general behaviour are ruled by <u>66heela</u>.

Cesta is an institution that can express already deeper mental states during treatment such as compliance, agitation or retardation that lead to treatment. *Acara* is ruling out when disturbances in the doshas and gunas influenced the person's behaviour into socially difficult manners. Aggressiveness, quarrel, disrespectfulness are plastering the person's way and society will leash back. Acara needs containment or it leads to profound suffering.

Rajas and Tamas are the gunas that affect (what in the west would be called) the mind. If they dominate, by pre-existing condition, impact or experiences like neglect, trauma, abuse or life style/ eating measures, mental disorders of insanity cloud the faculties of the mind, in particular the Buddhi. If Buddhi is affected, all the Samskaras continue In a perpetuate manner. The decision making capacity is not free of the previous tints of experience and therefore affecting the future in a particular way that inevitably leads to more pain. Wrong decision making affects all plains of life, it is inseparable from life.

Charaka's Aetiology of Unmada

Charaka categorises different causes and outcomes of the individual root of disturbance. In the following text, Charaka classifies and clarifies his observations. He defines aetiological factors, including digestion, spiritual and social aspects, emotional factors, self-responsibility and knowledge.Charaka explains the problems of wrong food choices and uncleanliness in lifestyle, words and choices.

Themes like insults to gods and higher family members are difficult to explain to the western mind. The neglect or absence of religious or spiritual thinking leads to an often discriminating view on Ayurveda medicine. If we look into the aspects of respect, we can probably understand that disrespectful behaviour causes problems. If someone needs to make decisions, always have to fight for everything, there is an absence of serenity if projects or relationship fail. And they tend to fail at some point.

Imagining life can be controlled is the outcome of a mind in hybris. Letting go of control, allowing influences to take over and step back from the results of our efforts are named mindfulness. Mindfulness is now even prescribed in the western medical system and paid by insurances. Western thinking embraces the rational mind but loses the concept of the irrational body.

Losing control leads to another cause of disease, which is fear. The principles of the Ayurveda diet are to be followed strictly to avoid the aggravation of the doshas. Every patient who was able to experience the change of diet was overwhelmed.

However, maintaining a freshly cooked diet in which certain foods cannot be mixed or consumed together is hard. Particularly if Buddhi has been disturbed cravings of certain foods often counteract all efforts in diet change, even if the person has already experienced the positive influence on their mental state. Poisoned food like preparations with milk and fruit, a huge amount of uncooked vegetables, cheese and other unsuitable combinations are often inhibiting sleep, positive thinking, proper digestion and appetite, happiness in positive body feelings and recovery.

Ayurveda and Yoga, used as Medicine and performed by experienced and professional therapists, could fill the demand for professional treatment of PTSD by introducing meaning-making skills and creating a safe space through controlled and supervised care and cooperation with the government. Both disciplines have provided immense expertise over the centuries.

However, a short weekend course focused on trauma-sensitive yoga or ayurveda, does not respect the mind of a trauma patient's multiple damages and needs, nor does it protect the practitioner themself. Practitioners and therapists need much longer, detailed, holistic and long-term supervised education in ayurveda and yoga to learn how to protect themselves and protect the patient.

This book aims to inquire if Yoga and Ayurveda are suitable methods to diagnose and treat trauma and possibly allow a more precise choice of which treatment method might be more successful in an individually tailored fashion.

Starting from the assumption that grief, sadness, anxiety and fear of pain are unavoidable, inevitably, they are part of life. Why do different human beings take other times to recover from trauma and develop different patterns to cope with stressful situations? Why do some individuals recover from stress and shock after a seriously prolonged time or even not at all? In contrast, some individuals show hardly any signs of distress after surviving even dramatic life events.

The following chapters on *unmada* and *cittodvega* attempt to prove that ancient Indian medicine named and described the changes in the mind and behaviour known as PTS/PTSD before western medicine discovered psychological disturbances in soldiers after World War I. Additionally, "The Yoga Sutras of Patanjali" describe how to observe the nature of the mind. They a deal with modifying and controlling the fluctuation of awareness between past and future *(buddhi, citta, manas).*

Analysing the benefits of holistic treatments like ayurveda with additional yoga practice, one must question the possibility of transferring ancient knowledge from millennia ago to modern patients' needs. Further examined, is it possible to achieve recovery, resilience or healing by taking single isolated parts out of context?

Some ayurvedic terms have already been misinterpreted and wrongly applied for many years. An important example is *ama*-removal treatments (*ama pacana*) marketed as "detox." There is re-labelling of traditional medical names going on, such as *unmada*, *cittodvega*, by reducing meaningful descriptive Sanskrit words and terms to western simplifications. Like PTSD, PTS, OBD and others name a collection of disturbances but do not consider the holistic view of recovery, resilience or healing options.

Ayurveda unfolds the full holistic richness of its healing tradition by following the rules of *dinacharya (daily regimen), vihara (lifestyle) and ahara* (nutrition). Ayurveda states that the best medicine is worthless without the proper nutrition and that nutrition is medicine or poison if not mastered. Yoga contributes to recovery and healing through developing mental stamina by achieving higher meaning-making goals.

The two sister traditions encourage indolence by developing knowledge of the self and purpose of life, however different their ways of achieving such and the deeper meaning might be.

For many individuals, global and situational meanings shatter after traumatic events. Both are definitions that describe the meaning-making model. Every

68

person has to reason one's behaviour, goals and feelings. Meaning-making represents a re-established and valued purpose of life and even the daily drive to get up. It defines social behaviour, standards and morals.

Ayurveda delivers concepts from individual perspectives of meaning to global meaning and from the kitchen to the poisonous medicine. It can restore meaning-making as it penetrates every aspect of life with its structure, knowledge and rituals. Once the rhythm of sleep and eating, exercise and recovery are re-established, the patient feels embedded into a care system and experiences its relaxing qualities in a safe space that travels with them.

Unmada and *Cittodvega*: **Ayurvedic Concepts of Psychiatry**

In his lecture on ayurvedic psychiatry, Prof. Ram Manohar states there is no ayurvedic psychology for the simple reason that one can study the mind only when it is not sane. (Ram Manohar, 2018). Body and mind are generally a tight-knit web and not divided in nature. They cannot be as different parts of a person; clearly, the psyche leaves the continuum. It shows signs of disturbance in case of insanity.

Ayurveda and yoga use empirical scientific tools to explore the patient's consciousness of the inner and outer world.

Everything about how:

- human consciousness works in terms of health or Unmada and Cittodvega
- attention is directed
- we get stuck in the past with our mind
- we travel in the future with our mind
- we avoid being in the present
- how to could achieve living in the present
- how to stay healthy
- reduce the impact of distress
- how to be respectful with literally everything that is around us—

Is explicitly described in Ayurveda in the Charaka Samhita, Ashtanga Hridaya, in the Sutras of Patanjali, the Gheranda Samhita, the Hatha Yoga Pradipika.

Ayurveda and yoga provide the knowledge to integrate stressful and devastating events in the faith and destiny of the patient to recover or even heal from those impacts over time. *Unmada* and *Cittovega* are the technical Sanskrit terms for clear definitions and descriptions of mental diseases, according to the classical scripture Ashtanga Hridaya and Charaka Samhita as well as the Bhutavidya. *Unmada* and *Cittodvega* translate as "madness" or "insanity".

There is a distinction between internal and external factors, including demons, that cause *Unmada* or *Cittovega*. Several texts in yogic and ayurvedic scriptures and philosophical and religious/ spiritual writings like the Mahabharata, the Upanishads, etc., describe or explain the function of the mind, memory and the law of desire, aversion and action (*karma*). They explain the various states of consciousness and how to master the challenges of emotions, find purpose and follow the rules and intuition.

Patanjali is considered the author of the "*Yoga Sutras*" which introduced the concept of the adverse mind and its misconception by introducing the term *klesha* into the discussion. Others, like the *Shiva Samhita, Hatha Yoga Pradipika* or the *Bhagavad Gita* from the *Mahabharata,* contain already precise descriptions of the function of the mind, the consciousness and how to master the mind and, therefore *karma*.

Karma is a widely misunderstood term and I will not enter a discussion about the different meanings in India and the western use nowadays. Just briefly said as *Karma* simply translates as action or that, which one does and takes responsibility for, it is often wrongly used in western countries as a term that describes punishment for wrongdoing (Karma will do the rest, a common Instagram post for describing the hope of "justice" however more closely to self-righteousness).

The western use clearly is influenced by Jewish Christian thinking of an almighty god who punishes the sinner. As the concepts of an almighty god or the concept of a sin are alien to the complex Hindu traditions, the term should be in the used in its simplicity here for better understanding of concepts of actions of the doshas, gunas and beyond.

These days "Trauma Yoga" or "Trauma-Sensitive Yoga" has been launched in the US and Europe. Any yoga in my understanding is by its very nature trauma-sensitive, as it is the claim of yoga to stop the fluctuations of the mind. (yoga citta vritti niruda) and therefore breaks the past-future movement of the mind (citta).

The modern claims for Trauma-sensitive yoga however, are that a focus on relaxation (instead of the general focus in the west on fitness) should allow the practitioner to heal from the stress of trauma. The classes offer techniques that follow western yoga standards (focus on asana and breathing) except that the students are selected for having reportedly survived a trauma incident in their life that still has an impact on their overall well-being or that they suffer from PTSD.

The yoga teachers might have special skills that they learned in special "Trauma-Sensitive—Yoga—Teacher—courses". In the US, those yoga courses are mostly packed with veterans from the Vietnam and Iraq wars (mostly of the same demographic group: male, white, over 50 years old, poly-toxic background); (Paola King, Trauma-Yoga teacher, San Francisco, US, 2020).

Yoga proves to master the ripples of the wandering mind (Patanjali Yoga Sutras, Samadhi—Pada, 1-4 The Purpose of yoga, cited translation by Nicholas Sutton, Oxford Centre for Hindu Studies). *Yoga citta-vritti-nirodhah* can possibly be understood as an invitation to dive into the yoga path in general.

However, by just taking bits of the yoga path and limiting it to a specific isolated problem (like Trauma-sensitive yoga, yoga for other ailments like MS, backpain—) that does not see the individuality of each patient but labels a complex issue with unlimited adaption patterns might not succeed on all levels of the injured being. Whatever had been hoped for when booking oneself into these classes could then lead to another frustrating experience. Feelings like being a failure, sadness, hopelessness and shame.

Yogic studies and the eight-fold path of *Patanjali* Yoga are designed to deeply penetrate consciousness concepts through dedicated, focused, intense self-practice and self-study. In the Chapter on **Pranayama—Treatment with Breathing,** some of the techniques are explained.

There is a hopeful perspective. Ayurveda governs precise guidelines for all and everything. Ayurveda is contributing to the treatment of *Unmada* and *Cittovega* through various distinct physical therapies, starting from *Dinacharya* (daily routine), *Dravyaguna* herbal therapy, *ahara-vihara* (lifestyle and nutrition), *shirodhara* (Olation of the forehead), *abhyanga* ("oil massage") to *Panc Karma (*The 5 Actions) to each individual's needs.

Ayurveda contributes to the specific understanding of the mind's distortion and how PTS and PTSD can develop in some individuals and some not. The concept of the *doshas* and their disturbances, accumulations and interactions with each other as well with the *gunas* (qualities of the mind), *manas* (the sensory motor mind), *citta* (the memory bank), the *ahamkara*, (I—ness) *and buddhi* (discriminative power)* are part of endless varieties of diseases described, diagnosed and accessible to treatment.

Yoga provides the technique to explore the self through self-inquiry, discipline, guidance and exercise of the *yamas* and *niyamas* (rules how to interact with the world and how to conduct oneself in the practice of yoga). On the other hand, there are the universe's rules, the unfolding of the *doshas* and *gunas*, the focus on well-being, balancing, nourishing what is empty and reducing what is stagnant or overfilled within Ayurveda.

Ayurveda is "the long-missed warm motherly hug," as most patients describe it. The warmth and care that re-establishes self-worth by feeling appreciated and looked after with care. Treatments with warm oil, simple healthy food and gentle touch often fill the inner void.

As one patient described it:—*as if you find an inner living being inside yourself that is worth to live for, that needs to be loved. It is maybe your inner child that you discover. It is still there. It is wonderful*! (Patient M. W., Psychoanalyst, 2019)

Ayurveda displays an enormous range of different treatments—from nourishing *(brahmana)*, to reducing *(langhana and shodhana)*, from restoring *(rasayana and shamana),* to eliminating *(Amapacana).*

The different applications of medicated oil (such as *brahmi thail, ashvagandha taila, karpuradi kuzhampo, anu taila)* as in *shirodhara, abhyanga, bhasti, nasya* are just a tiny part of it and are widely used in the west.

The vast number of active pharmaceutical plants, animal products, mineral preparation (*dravyaguna*) and pharmacopeia of toxicology (*rasaushadhi*) are not understood and tested in randomised studies. There are uncountable variations of medical prescriptions in India, based on so many different climates, sources, races and tribes and hundreds of cultures and languages. India's ancient scientific medical and philosophical traditions might reveal even more options for resilience, recovery and healing through medical treatment that is currently known.

The heart of ayurvedic treatments, not only for physical ailments in general but also for psychiatric diseases, is the *Panc Karma* treatment. *Panc Karma*

---

* translation of the Sanskrit terms of concepts from: Yoga and Psychotherapy, The Evolution of Consciousness, Swami Rama.

combines various eliminating procedures like vomiting, elimination through the intestine, the nose, etc. *Panc arma* is considered a reset of the body and the mind. It allows the patient to reconnect with their body through an intense experience and the removal of *Ama*, physical and mental *Ama* likewise. (Prof. Ram Manohar, in a private meeting, Birstein, Rosenberg Academy, 2019)

Charaka: The Cause of Unmada

Unmada, a major mental disorder, has been known to ayurvedic practitioners since ancient times in India. Yet, in the Vedic period, the disease was thought to be caused due to Grahas/demons, as a disease that affects a vulnerable person but still has it's origin outside but in Ayurveda it is considered a major mental illness. Yet when we look into traumatic injuries, we do see the exogenic factor as well as the adaption of the individual, which can vary from hyper reaction to hypo-reaction, from recovery to drug abuse.

Unmada describes more a quality and a state of mind and awareness, not a disease. The symptoms vary from what would be nowadays diagnosed as a psychotic disorder, ego-state, schizophrenia, manic psychosis or as depressive disorders.

Signs and symptoms of *Unmada* according to Charaka Samhita, Sharma, according to Das interpretation from 2000. He writes about the Intellectual confusion displayed incoherent speech or unsteady vision, A sensation of a vacuum in the heart is often described by patients and well known already at Charaka's time. (vacant mindedness). If the patient is struck by Unmada, he is unable to experience appropriate experiences of pleasure or sorrow and loses the peace of mind.in fact, the mind wavers.

A text by Charaka gives a clear insight into ayurvedic thinking. It describes how the mind gets altered by stress—and mentions a factor of mental function described as dissociation in modern western terms. The expression "the vacuum in the heart" clearly refers to this. It represents the loss of contact with the self, personal individual desires and needs.

Consequently, there will be no meaningful decision or action following, as the analysis of the moment is clouded by misconception of the NOW or even completely disrupted (dissociation).The following text explains Charaka's insights on the possible causes of insanity. It illustrates the changes and respective non—changes of the victim's or patient's perception of reality and the adapting lifestyle. Brief modern explanations were added as interpretative comments.

According to Ayurveda, digestion in the term of Agni is the source and the cause of health or disease (*bhoga rhoga* yoga). Wrong food choices are the fundamental factor for diseases. Modern descriptions of *dosha* aggravation and *dhatu* ("tissue") high blood pressure, depression, high triglycerides and infertility are amongst other, even life-threatening consequences of wrong food choices. Individuals can make bad food choices, not knowing their individual needs, yet the modern food industry encourages them.

Charaka mentions "polluted food". Polluted food causes short or even long-lasting unwanted effects. Pollution refers to fertilizers, germs, industrial herbicides and contaminated food. Substantially, alcohol is poison and considered contaminated food, too. It is rotten fermented and its effects are narcotic, painkilling, headache-inducing, nausea, euphoria, depression and addiction.

Being disrespectful to the elderly, teachers and influential people is quite common among young people. Aristotle said: "This young generation is the worst ever!" There is a big difference between Asian and western societies: A project named: "Breaking the Rules" turned out to have very different answers: while westerners had no problems of imaging how to break the rules, Asians took a while to understand and picture something.

Westerners came up with selfish and ungenuine or meaning-making attempts, like smashing a window, having three partners at a time, robbing a bank, etc. Their ideas of breaking the rules were mostly against common social rules but were given individual benefits and considered fun things to do. The attitude was elation and mischievous.

Asian people, however, were thinking: "how sad," anti-social and disrespectful it would be breaking the rules. It would disgrace the family. Breaking the rules was considered a loss in value and not as fun. The same attitude came with bad school results: westerners worried about their future start after a bad exam, Asian's concern was about upsetting their mothers.

A Patient with a long history of self-inquiry wrote: "What does it mean: breaking the rules? It means that I have had the courage to make something happen. I feel scared of breaking rules around bureaucracy. I've adventured out in many ways and have felt that I broke the rules by not believing in them. The older I've gotten I've started to believe in many more rules, like here in Germany.

74

I have to be followed more rules (—) to break the rules to me means standing up for what was right. If I break the rules, it is with good reason! If I break the rules, it is because that rule does not align with me and my truth (—)". (Patient T, 5/2020)

While happiness exists in all cultures, It's meaning and the way it's experienced vary enormously: Happiness Around the World: The Paradox of Happy Peasants and Miserable Millionaires, 2020.

Interpretation of the Four Causative Factors According to Charaka

The causative factors one and two are of little interest in understanding PTSD or PTS. Although factor one can be considered a supportive factor in the development of distress, yet can slow down recovery. The second factor needs to look at how it could translate into western understanding.

If an instruction follows only partially, it is useless and harmful. Charaka states: do not treat the patient who cannot follow instructions. They are most likely to harm the reputation of the *vaidya*, interrupt their healing process and even keep others away from help by giving them a bad reputation. Exploring the causative factor 3 is the main factor in understanding Charaka's concept of trauma.

Fear affects the heart (*hridaya*) through the rise of the *doshas*. The heart is the centre of intellectual activities and emotions. Often the heart is considered the seat of the mind, not so in the original texts. *Hridaya* gets disturbed by the increase in the *doshas*. In its function as a steady and adaptable blood pump, the heart is vulnerable to emotional disturbances, fear and anxiety in particular. Fear and anxiety can also be known as distress.

The blood supply is disturbed in those vessels responsible for carrying the mental stimuli to the different parts of the body. Vasoconstriction, inability to fight or flight, angina pectoris, high or extremely low blood pressure, an increase in heart rate or even Broken-Heart-Syndrome are the current terms for a blockage of the *srotas*.

Even years after the initial shock or traumatic event, it is still possible to detect those parameters by simply measuring the vital factors in case of arousal. These bio-medical factors are necessary to monitor as they are easily accessible. Often a drastic increase of the pulse rate during a consultation (in case of traumatic arousal around 140 beats/min and higher), shakiness, hyperventilation—

with dropping of blood oxygen, increase or decrease of blood sugar and cortisol levels are used to monitor the effects and progress of the treatment in general.

Although not all patients show such clear signs, it is worthwhile to incorporate regular check-ups of vital parameters like BP, Cardiac Echo, 24-hour Blood Pressure measurement and blood oxygenation in the Ayurveda or Yoga consultation. In the longer run, Pro-Lactin, Cortisol, blood sugar and Thyroid (Hashimoto antibodies) should incorporate into a regular check-up.

Constant distress affects cognitive ability. Diagnosis of Awareness Deficiency Disorder (ADD) or ADHS in children are post-traumatic stress disorder related and cognitive disturbances. Gabor Mate is leading to understanding ADD as a part of a traumatic injury.

The mind cannot be peaceful and focused when fear and anxiety disrupt the flow of the *doshas*. The mental activity loses its capacity to be open and receive impressions from the outside and the inside. If a traumatic injury has happened, the mind clouds memories and fear of repetition.

The following source of Charaka Samhita with commentaries from Bhagwan Dash continues to explain the symptoms and signs of an afflicted heart:

The above is a similar description of a traumatised patient, including a detailed description of episodes of dissociation.

Unmada: The Inner and Outer Treatment Decisions Made by Discovering the Root

Charaka not only defines causative factors but gives detailed guidelines about treatment choices. The treatments vary from the root cause of the mental disturbance. In western psychiatry, the same medication given is merely SSRI (Serotonin). No selective guideline refers to the patients' cause of suffering.

Charaka differentiates *Unmada* into four causative factors: *agantu* (exogenous) and *nijottha* (endogenous). The proposed treatments then vary according to the detection of the specific god or demon attacking the patient's mind or identifying the various kinds of *dosha* aggravation. Treatments are specific from medicated ghee to rituals or mantras, home and specific nutritional food. The physician or *vaidya* should not beat the patient.

In severe *Unmada*, where symptoms are contradictory, the doctor should refrain from any treatment at all. Therefore, all treatments would contradict the other and worsen the patient's condition. Translated into western psychiatric terms: severe *Unmada* could describe patients displaying borderline syndrome, multiple personalities—discussed as a post-traumatic stress disorder or patients with bipolar disorder.

A closer look into disease description in Ayurveda reveals more qualification and specification of illness than the general idea that it is either "*vata, pitta* or *kapha.*" The complexity of understanding the human organism, functions, influence of the mind while ill, environmental and causative factors date back thousands of years.

As therapists we are differentiating not only the differences in the aggravated doshas, but the gunas, the Dhatus (tissue related), Srotas (connecting vessel related), Malas (excrement related) and more planes of diagnose. However, there is no symptom or cause, no change at all that is not influencing, affecting, changing the whole. Connection and changing the field of connection is the fundamental empiric experience of Ayurveda and Yoga that make them so different to the western allopathic linear thinking.

Aetiology, Signs and Symptoms of *Vatika Unmada*:

Vata represents movement and any instability in lifestyle or diet lets it aggravated. Cold food, skipping meals, too little food as well as emotions like worry, passion or anxiety lead to the state Vatika Unmada. Charaka mentions weeping, laughing, dancing, speaking or moving limbs in an inappropriate place or at inappropriate times as a clear sign. The skin is rough and often reddish purple.

Aetiology, Signs and Symptoms of *Paittika Unmada*

Described is a heated personality that tends to feel and express anger, aggression, irritability. The person is fiery in arguments and tends to overrun people with their impatience.

Aetiology, Signs and Symptoms of *Kaphaja Unmada*

Sluggishness and laziness, depression and a whitish or decoloured complexion to the skin describe kaphaja. The malnutrition can be represented by overweight, wrong food choices for cold, oily, carbohydrate rich food.

Consumption and hoarding are the main issues. The person wants to be left alone or gathers people around her. Messy lifestyle is represented through stickiness as a key symptom.

The psychological trauma was already described thousands of years ago. Charaka has given strict limitations to the treatment of certain psychological disorders.

In the presented research, more symptoms are named, including the empirical analysis of treatment and management of psychological problems following traumatic injuries.

Sattva	*Rajas*	*Tamas*
Pacifying, enlighten	Dynamic, forward striving	Static, inhibition
Striving for knowledge and understanding	Pain and pleasure bound	fatigue of sense organs, easy losing sensorial interest and connection
Clean, tidy	On the move	agnostic
Spiritually grounded	Fanatic, clinging to ideas	inactive
Honesty	egoistic	poor
Correct behaviour rooted in authenticity	reacting	Craving for sleep
gratitude	Irritable, easily startled, pain	Worried for no cause, not changing
Excellent and correct memory. buddhi	Narcissistic traits, dominant	Erratic behaviour
prompt to learn from observation, serious studying and listening	learns for dominance and power	Does not like to learn or improve
Demonstrating authenticity, respect and values	Brave, straight forward	Obsolescent to change
Supportive	greedy	Sticky, clinging, respectless
helper	cruel	stubborn
benevolent	tense	Due to no engagement

Behavioural and Psychological Manifestation of Triguna, summary from Charaka's observations Important Ayurveda Texts for the Research of the Treatment of Trauma in Ayurveda.

In the Charakasamhita, the risk factors for *Unmada* include *Bhirunam*— those lacking courage, a weak mind and *Upaklistasattvanam*—those afflicted by the stress of the mind.

The eighth chapter of *Nidanasthana* of Charaka, points out that the leading causes of *Unmada* are fear, shock and sorrow— *bhayatrasashokairunmadaapasmaaraanaam*—related to the modern concept of post-traumatic stress disorder.

It is also clearly mentioned in chapter seven of *Nidanasthana* of *Charakasamhita* that *Unmada* is caused by the mind afflicted (*abhyahata*) by *abhighata* (trauma) due to emotionally distressing experiences. Thus, the psychological impact of emotionally disturbing experiences in life can lead to *Unmada* as described in ayurvedic texts, providing insight into PTSD from an ayurvedic perspective.

Dating back thousands of years, ayurvedic researchers, doctors and rishis have been able to identify such complex behavioural, emotional and physical change after a shock and then treat it successfully over centuries accordingly. The treatment has always been multi-dimensional, often involving diet and lifestyle as much as psycho-spiritual practices simultaneously and embedded in a whole concept of procedures starting with *dinacharya* (daily routine) to religious rituals.

The cause of the disease does not need to be labelled. The effects and treatments are significant. Ayurveda has not developed a complex theory in which the specific reason of *Unmada* and its understanding are essential to overcoming the symptoms. Rituals are the primary routine for treatment. Routines turn into rituals.

A patient G. once mentioned that: "—addiction is a great way to structure the day because it is routine as well as ritual."

Patients who suffer from addiction and traumatic injuries have been the major clients at the Society of Friends, Berlin. Substance abuse and addiction often jeopardises all effort as the addict defines almost all aspects of life under addiction. Losing one's wealth, beauty, social standard, friends and family and even one's life is often the way and seems to be less frightening than living in a world of pain without meaning. The addict usually follows instructions. If partially followed, the instruction is useless and can become harmful.

As Charaka states: "do not treat the patient who cannot follow instructions." The patient is most likely to harm the reputation of the *Vaidya*, interrupt their healing process, jeopardise it and even keep others away from help by having a bad reputation. However, this book will encourage therapists to dive into classical Ayurveda and experience a significant in behaviour, goals in life, self-care and therefore perspective in life.

Unmada—Analysing the Concepts of Mental Insanity in Ayurvedic Texts

Peter Levine states that Trauma impact shocks the brain, the mind gets on hold and the body freezes in shock. It is an overwhelming unfortunate event or a chain of events that hurls the victim in a raging sea of torment, helplessness and fear.

Unmada: The Inner and Outer Treatment Decisions—Discovering the Root

Charaka not only defines causative factors but gives detailed guidelines about treatment choices. The treatments vary according to the root of course of the mental disturbance. In western psychiatry, the same medication is merely SSRI. No selective guideline refers to the patients' cause of suffering.

Charaka differentiates *Unmada* into four causative factors: *agantu* (exogenous) and *nijottha* (endogenous). The proposed treatments then vary according to the detection of the specific god or demon attacking the patient's mind or identifying the various kinds of *dosha* aggravation. Treatments are specific from medicated ghee to rituals or *mantra* (religious/spiritual recitation), *homa* (spiritual fire ceremony) and particular nutritional food. The physician (*vaidya*) should not pressure the patient.

In severe *unmada*, all symptoms are contradictory. It is advised (the old scriptures) that the doctor refrains from any treatment. Therefore, all treatments would contradict the other and worsen the patient's condition. Translated into western psychiatric terms: severe *Unmada* describes patients displaying

80

borderline syndrome, multiple personalities, post-traumatic stress disorder or patients with bipolar disorder.

Further Classifications of Disease According to Charaka

Classifications and terms of diseases and their prognosis from Charaka Samhita, Vimana Sthana, Chapter 6, Verse 4. Charaka not only defines health or the onset of disease but delivers measurements for prognosis, called Prabhava Bheda.

Sadhya: the condition can be healable—
Divided into:
Sukha Sadhya (easy to heal)
Kricchra Sadhya (difficult to heal)
Asadhya (cannot be cured)
Intensity: *Bala Bheda*
Mild (*mrudu*), severe (*daruna*)
Location: *adhishthana*
Body (*sharira adhishthana*)
Mind—*citta, manas, buddhi* (*mano adhishthana*)
Nature of Causative Factors: *Nimitta Bheda*
Endogenous (*sva-dhatu-vaishamaya*)
Exogenous (*agantu nimitta*)
Based on the Site of Origin: *Ashaya Bheda*
Stomach (*amashaya*)
Colon (*pakvashaya samuttha*)
Mind/psyche in the sense of *rajasika* or *tamasika*
All diseases are either only one or all the different categories.

Causes of Certain Incurable Diseases:

Ayurveda never claimed there would cure for every ailment or discomfort. In the west, most people doubt natural medicine can be helpful at all although there is a growing community that believes in natural medicine but often applies it as how they were used to do with allopathic medicine: take them when the problem is there, in large amounts. Rejecting help from allopathic biomedical medical help can be often seen these days as the modern medicine is losing trust.

There is, however, an unrealistic hope that Ayurveda could simply heal anything. If Ayurveda does not help, then the patient is to blame. Unfortunately, the attitude to blame the victim when they are not recovering, as expected, is the rule and not the exception.

The Curable and the Incurable

Further chapters of the textbook Charaka Samhita lighten up the specific conditions with a realistic way of resilience; recovery or healing could be possible.

After defining curable diseases, there are factors that inhibit healing. As therapists, we often remain helpless if the patient is continuing harmful behaviour or attitudes, even if knowing better. An important factor in treating or even healing the patient is not only to have a proper experienced concept, but to take the patient and one's own capabilities into consideration.

The lack of compliance in the sense of proper attendance and equipment of the patient is named as number one. This includes a lack of financial resources as well as problems in distance to the treatment facilities, problems in the family and housing. A lack of self-control hinders the patient to attain the treatments, to follow in instructions and to demonstrate continuity in the requirements of treatment. Addiction, laziness, excuses havoc the best treatment.

However, not only the patients' issues can stop the healing but incompetent physicians were already pointed at in the Charaka. A lack of proper treatment facilities and options due to the complexity of the disease including the surrounding of the victim (like in case of trauma from domestic abuse, the author) inhibit healing processes from the root.

Learning and studying Ayurveda in the west is now possible and these days even easy accessible through online options, yet it is not easy to find quality immediately and a teacher, Guru, Professor who's qualifications meet the authentic ayurvedic requirements for profound diagnose and healing and is capable or willing to connect with the students and theory of individual needs. In the past century, traveling to India for Ayurveda studies meant being at least fluent in Sanskrit and another local language.

These days, it's weekend trips for Yoga Teacher Training. It is necessary to control westerners' hunger for Ayurveda therapy to maintain high-quality standards. Supervision is an option for psychoanalytical working psychologists but not necessarily the gold standard.

For ayurvedic practitioners in Germany, there is no obligatory supervision. There is a lifelong web of supportive mentorship in India after students finish their exams. The individualisation in western societies reflects in the western medical system just the same way: the freshly accredited doctor or medical person starts practicing right away but does not necessarily have a supervisor, a mentor or obligations for further educational studies.

In alternative healing, it is even worse: most seminars end with a certificate of attendance but not with an apprenticeship. In my eyes only an apprenticeship is a reliable tool in education. Apprenticeships are the exception, although it would help increase the standard of education and reduce the cost of therapy.

In my clinic, I was running a 40 patient/day practice only with the help of 8 apprentices. their questions, their observations, their backgrounds made it possible to review each and every step of treatments that I thought could be taken for granted. I employed apprentices from Japan, Switzerland, Latvia, Martinique, Colombia, Brazil, Russia, Syria, Afghanistan, Iran, India, US (California), Greece, Nigeria, Serbia, UK, Austria, Australia, Netherlands and other countries. Each of them brought in their tremendously rich cultural background and taught all of us the subtle or bigger stepping stones to avoid in intercultural context.

Diseases are Innumerable—The Sources of Structure in Ayurveda
The Psychic *Doshas*: *Mano-Dosha*

A closer look into the *Mano-Dosha* classification leads to discovering the surprisingly accurate description of the different states of mind written down and categorised thousands of years ago. Modern psychiatry has tried to explain the function of the mind since the 1800s. Explanations of trauma only began within the last 40 years. It is nothing but impressive how detailed in classification and description the old ayurvedic and yoga textbooks are. The data was found through dedicated practice, observation and evaluation of numerous patients and students.

The value of empirical study is underestimated chiefly in the west. If the effect is not measured by physics or chemistry, it is often not scientific.

Mano-Dosha: The Mind, The Spirit, The Innermost Core

The state of a *sattvic* mind (contentment, autonomy, own sets of desires and dreams, encouraging growth, not controlling, equilibrium, etc.) does not emerge as an explanation in the context of disease. Only *rajas* and *tamas* are the types that cause morbidity. *Sattva* is a psycho-physiological factor, whereas *tamas* and *rajas* are psycho-pathological factors. While *sattva* cannot cause any psychopathological behaviour or emotion, *rajas* and *tamas* do so.

Charaka is further differentiating the emotions that stem from the *Mano-Doshas* as:

Kama (lust)
Krodha (anger)
Lobha (greed)
Moha (attachment)
Irshya (envy)
Mana (ego)
Mada (pride)
Shoka (depression)
Cinta (worry)
Udvega (anxiety)
Bhaya (fear)
Harsha (excitement)

The physiological *dosha* activity allows all emotions to unfold freely without constraint, yet with equilibrium and contentment. The mental aspects of *doshas* often combine with the mental *gunas*.

Gunas in ayurveda and yoga, although both originate in the *Samkhya* philosophy system, cannot be understood as similar in meaning and, consequently, in action. The mental *gunas* in ayurveda are different aspects of mental activity and dominantly inherited and acquired factors. Unlike the *dosha* as in the constitution (*prakriti*), which surrenders under universal laws but allows making own choices (*vikriti*), the *gunas* can be controlled and developed.

A life lived according to the eternal rules of the universe and with the good fortune of all aspects of life allows the person to unfold his full potential, maintaining good health and joyful life. Yet life cannot be controlled by our best wishes and loss, grief or shock will eventually happen, even to the luckiest ones.

Suppose the *doshas* get disturbed or aggravated by wrong food choices, environment, activity or even the *gunas rajas* or *tamas* (unfortunate accumulation of emotions). The state of mind and health needs to be carefully restored into balance. Feelings change the activity of the mind. The mind can change the action of the *doshas*. The change of balance in the *doshas* can change the *gunas'* dominance.

Envy, anger and sadness do not cause illness immediately. If they become predominant or a permanent state of mind, fixed emotions will cause distress. Distress leads to changes in the *doshas*. Under the influence of anguish, the person is more likely to make wrong choices, lack discipline or the *dinacharya*; the daily routine gets disturbed. This is not only the case where emotions like sadness or anger are dominant; however, the same is valid for prolonged and intense happiness.

Yet, western research does not inquire about happiness, thrill and excessive joy as ill causative factors. Too much happiness can lead to careless, lusty behaviour that does not respect the individual's physical limitations. Again, if the state of happiness is not a permanent ecstasy, like occurring in the first stage of falling in love, there is nothing wrong with happiness. Happiness is a feeling of contentment, satisfaction and freedom of longing, lust or needs and mental or physical distractions are the best sign of health.

The endless cycle of various emotions that come to the surface of our consciousness are healthy *guna/dosha* relations. Controlling, guiding and cultivating them determines individual faith.

Translating *guna* and *dosha* as mind (*guna*) and body (*dosha*) relevant categories would not respect the detailed descriptions from ayurveda and yoga of the different fractions of our consciousness, memory, instincts and decision-making parts of the brain. The terminology is not a "term to term" translation but needs an interpretation of the whole socio-cultural history.

Buddhism and Islam have also contributed to the richness of ayurveda and yoga with their very own and unique concepts. The Vedic-influenced cultural background is the most accessible and studied in the west.

As the word Veda in ayurveda is mentioned in Charaka from the root Vid. Sushruta, the medical textbook author for surgery, uses the root Vid in the sense of: to attain. Ayu is mostly translated as life; however, the meaning is the span from the beginning of life to its end, which clearly differs in the context of medicine and philosophy. If we look at life's dynamic states, it's intelligence and happiness then we can understand it as a continuum form the very source in the universe to its journey of consciousness.

Any disturbance or circumstance that interrupts the process, the mind gets seriously affected and the intellect loses its balance. The doshas aggravated and vitiated enter the cardiac region and obstruct the channels of the mind, resulting in insanity. It is a detailed and exact description of a person suffering from a post-traumatic disorder, long before a single phenomenon of mental illness has been acknowledged or described in the west.

1. When an individual is timid

Being timid in the sense of Unmada is probably not a correct and direct translation. The term "hiding or suffering from anxiety" or "agoraphobia" as in public or sociophobia would be another interpretation.

2. When the mind is afflicted by the predominance of Rajas and Tamas

If *rajas* and *tamas* dominate the mind, it becomes inner restlessness with no way out. The mind is dull while moving in circles, without apparent thought and desire. No plan can spark light and introduce changes. There is no outcome, no direction, but mentally the person experiences frustration and anger. A modern term would be ADD (Awareness Deficiency Disorder), where the patient cannot concentrate on a single subject at a time yet has enough energy to achieve the goal.

Instead, the person starts getting tired. Some patients take disproportional naptimes that drastically interfere with their work hours. Procrastination is another example. The work becomes postponed due to a lack of clarity, motivation and inner inhibition. Procrastination connects to self-worth and even narcissism. Narcissism is often a symptom of the injured soul.

It reflects a feeling of superiority (an attempt to prevent further damages) and an inner void and doubts covered up with arrogance. The person cannot experience a setback in their work by not getting the best result. The tamasic attitude stops the patient from benefiting from an acknowledgment by delivering work in a last-minute mode. A job done under the deadline threat is never as good as well-thought-out work. Frustration and anger are the results of not even finishing the work.

Narcissistic adults emotionally abandoned by their caretakers show low self-esteem and self-damaging behaviour. However, not all procrastinators are traumatised people. Traumatised people have a much higher rate of procrastinating due to learned avoidance mechanisms.

3. *When doshas in the body are aggravated and vitiated*

Ayurveda describes precisely different stages of disease development, called *shat kriya kala*. It explains where illness originates and manifests clearly step by step. Accordingly, in the case of illness, these steps show the withdrawal of pathogenic factors in the body.

While the first three subclinical stages are often not detected, *sancaya*, *prakopa and prasara*, the later, named, *sthanasamsraya*, *yyakti* and *bheda* are clinical stages of the pathogenesis. The stages allow proper diagnosis as well as prognosis of the unfolding of further complications.

- *Sancaya*—(natural accumulation of *doshas)*

Sancaya means the accumulation of the *doshas* in their natural sites, for instance, Vata doshas's seat in the pelvic region and the bones, Pitta dosha reigns from the area of the diaphragm in the middle of the abdomen, Kapha dosha sits in the upper chest and throat.

- *Prakopa* (more accumulation)

—if dosha aggravating factors are influencing the person on any level, accumulation occurs. At this stage, there is still simple correction possible by eliminating the causative factors.

- *Prasara*—(overflow)

Prasara means "spreading, expanding." Other parts of the body, organs or systems of the body are affected in all directions. *Prasara* can involve *Rakta* as a dhatu (tissue) and all of three *doshas*.

- *Sthanasamshraya*—(disease augmentation)

The pathogenic factors localised in one place become damaged (vitiated *doshas* with *dushyas* or local tissues). The actual disease occurs and is associated with the appearance of prodromal symptoms.

—*Vyakti* Manifestation—

The manifestations of signs and symptoms of an acute disease. This is mostly the time when the patient shows up for treatment, as the symptoms are disturbing their overall wellbeing.

—*Bheda* Complications—

At this stage the disease becomes acute, chronic or already had moved into the field of being incurable because extensive damage sustained or irreversible structural change happened if the untreated condition is at the stage of *vyakti*.

Shat Kriya Kala is the knowledge to detect illnesses and enables them to perform the right treatment before incurable damage is manifested. In western alternative medicine/complementary medicine we describe this still as prevention of disease; however, there might be already symptoms discovered (like catching cold easily, sleep disturbances—etc). In ayurveda at this stage there would preferable Panc karma therapy performed to reset and cure at early stages.

The ayurveda concept of *Ahara* is the core of health: everything should be digested fully. Digestion is a complex process, starting with seeing and smelling the object (our taste buds are active just by seeing a food, as the lemon test proves.

Just mentioning: I am going to bite in a juicy lemon, provides a particular combination of saliva juices immediately), tasting it, swallowing, breaking it down, absorbing it and eliminating it. Absorption and elimination are fascinating parts of a holistic diagnosis. They can vary so much from person to person and from the food choice that is made. Food choices are often misunderstood as: the body asks for it's needed.

According to ayurveda, the food choice rather displays the imbalances of the doshas. A Vata disturbance asks for more Vata, however much the inner quest for the opposite is there. Pitta often comes up with excuses: I deserve that, Kapha is convinced: my body tells me, I should that ayurveda can detect imbalances before making the wrong food choice or unknowingly suffer from malnutrition because of incomplete digestion and absorption.

Charaka continues to explain problems in healing. *When the body is exceedingly depleted or is in a state bad health due to other diseases.*

Inadequate or poor food intake, wrong food combinations, without willing to change, excessive exercise or physical straining work particularly after 6 pm, late exercising, too little recovery time, lack of deep sleep, childbirth, breastfeeding, blood loss, accidents, overuse of recreational drugs, etc., might postpone a holistic treatment. Patience is required with sensitive guidance and education to keep the patient motivated.

Other chronic or consumptive diseases can stop the patient from the path to recovery.

If we have a closer look into the trauma—disease connection we will find that a constant exposure to stress (that can be current, like in narcissistic relationships, narcissistic parenting, ill family members or work situations or unhealed trauma) leads easily to reoccurring health problems. On the other hand, some severe health issues might come up front, like cancer, injuries that might need primary attention and the trauma healing might feel less urgent.

However, stress is always related to an increase of stress hormones that block healing efforts. Keeping the patient motivated and addressing other health issues might lead to some disappointment. However, life-threatening health issues might have to be targeted first help to decrease the symptoms. Once the physical health is improving, deep trauma healing can proceed and emotional balance can be restored.

Missing a time frame for surgical intervention in case of cancer or other necessary treatments can be, in my experience, a life threatening mistake. The example of a breast cancer patient who was advised by an alternative healer to solve the traumatic stress from a suspected rape in childhood first, as it would be the only road to healing and then start chemo and operation, would have probably led to a fatal end.

Charaka then focuses on the mind or, better, the mental state of the patient. When the mental gunas are afflicted over and over again by passion, anger, greed, excitement, fear, attachment, exertion, anxiety and grief an emotional rollercoaster personality is an inhibiting factor in recovery so is emotional instability and disturbance with high responsiveness to distress often the leading symptom of PTSD.

Now: Where to start?

Careful guidance in effect control helps the patient to avoid situations that could be harmful. In western psychiatry, diagnosis like Borderline Personality Disorder, Bipolar (manic-Depressive) Personality Disorder, Compulsive Behaviour Disorder, Histrionic Personality Disorder, Awareness Deficiency Syndrome are examples for their diagnostic tools to decide treatment options to help navigate through pain, neglect and distress.

The victim's mind has lost its ability to move from distress to equilibrium and shows either an absence of emotions and the opposite: an overly emotional behaviour. The intense highs and lows often create an ecstatic feeling of being alive. One patient remarked: "—even if I am on my knees and howling in the dark, thinking, that is it, enough, even than in my darkest moments I feel more alive than in the mediocracy of meaningless conversations, the stupidity of work talk or relationship hugging!"

Even experiencing terrible emotional arousals can release a cascade of hormones similar to falling in love. The physical part responsive to endocrinal levels can stimulate a cocktail of chemical neuroactive substances that can create an addictive response in itself. An increase in heartbeat rate, widening pupils and increased blood circulation in the limbs due to a high sympathetic (*rajas-pitta*) response are signs of distress (examples are the paradox emotional responses of a person getting married as well as the loss of a loved one, severe injury, chronic terminal diseases or even childbirth).

These symptoms are addictive in themselves as they hit the dopamine response. The silence after arousal is 'magnificent', as one patient named it. It is necessary to explain the shift of emotional response as they might feel lifeless and suicidal at some point and immediately after feel hyperactive, attractive or lovable.

Patients can become used to being depressed that they might oversee moments that are tragic in general and that depression is a healthy response to those stressful events. They might be judged as unable to respond to grief, loss or other sad moments adequately and seen as lacking empathy or being awkward.

A traumatised patient has not received an impregnation against every other miserable feeling of loss and grief however, the general overload with pain and feeling disconnected can lead to a frozen response to new traumatic events. One patient had described it as ana anaesthesia to livelihood. They might not notice that their feeling could be even a healthy response to a new outside stress factor.

As Greta said during Corona Virus lockdown: "*I am so miserable. I am so sad, I don't understand why people are sad when nothing is changing from sadness to sadness.*"

Depression or better melancholy, if it is limited to a certain time and under control can be considered a healthy response to threatening and unclear external situations and is not a disease that needs treatment per se. Grieving after loss is a healthy response. Adaption to an unhealthy environment is not a sign of health, more likely a survival attempt of a traumatised person.

Charaka did not stop here but shares his observations on people who were exposed to excessive physical assault. During ongoing physical assaults, healing cannot take place. A safe space needs establishment first.

Charaka continues to point out that insanity that stems from assault ends in a perversion of the mind or intellect Insanity is characterised by the perversion of the manas, buddhi, citta consciousness, affects learning, knowledge, memory, desire and manners as we have seen earlier.

Further he rolls out and it is such a concrete and profound description what happens to the survivor: *the* patient either does not remember anything or remembers things incorrectly due to the confusion of the faculties of the mind. The patient then gets involved in unpleasant and undesirable activities that lead to more pain and confusion. We can clearly draw a line here to the observation of a high percentage of comorbidity in traumatised patients, such as drug addiction, etc.

Conclusion: The Perfect Jeweller

Charaka has created a universal outline for the diagnosis of insanity as it displays in PTSD. In his concept of *Unmada,* there are detailed descriptions of the different causative factors. Insanity (*Unmada*) resulting from psychological trauma should be treated differently than the diseases described in Kayachikitsa or Shalakya Tantra. He had clearly defined a psychological approach to understanding the various shatters of the patient's memories.

P. Levine points out that there is confusion about the role of memory in the pathology of trauma and its role in the healing process as well. The discoveries done so far a clearly contradicting each other. This leads to misapplication of therapeutic techniques, he adds disappointedly.

As long as survivors of traumatic events are doubted as they seem to be unable to remember correctly what happened, where, when, with whom etc.

without taking in consideration that the brain shuts down during stressful events, for instance, as it is busy trying to find escape routes, there will be no way out of the distress.

The memory should not be taken as a proof and the content of the memory as a tool to understand the impact as it is not accurate for the above reasons. The absence of even the confused memory can be more likely taken as a measure to what extent the damage had been done. Particularly survivors of sudden impact, like suicide bombing or attacks out of the blue, often cannot recall the before and after clearly.

Survivors of domestic abuse are often in co-dependent relationships or, as children, are in fully depending relationships with the abuser and cannot differentiate between their actions or the abusers action. They also often have been told to forget the incident and were often threatened to experience further harm if they would reach out for hep or tell other people about the "incident".

So, memory therefore cannot an indicator to understand the truth of trauma as the memory is not an objective storage of information as we will also see later in this book—

Charaka has given explanations and descriptions of the complex symptoms and signs that come with insanity as Unmada and has outlined treatment precise guidelines as well. He emphasises the best and special education of the therapist as the most important factor! Ayurveda, therefore, offers through the ancient knowledge of Charaka a complete compendium of appliable techniques, empirical knowledge and definitive herbal and physical therapies.

Different from western approaches, where the patient has to fit into the treatment methods, ayurveda offers a treatment approach that validates the individual constitution, the experiences, the nutrition, the lifestyle and the abilities of the patient. It then tailors a perfect treatment plan which incorporates meaning-making and universal approaches.

The restoration of the patients' inner landscape and their ability to restore *connection* rather than suppressing symptoms or treating the symptoms resulting from adaption to the sad and unwanted memory fixation is possible with proper diagnosis, treatment plans and adequate treatments. The whole concept delivers hundreds of treatment options that re-establish the patient's connectedness to the world, release unwanted PTSD symptoms and prevent further and possible future damage through self-inquiry (not including natural disasters, criminal acts, diseases).

Charaka has a holistic approach. As said: *"The perfect jeweller is making the jewellery according to the stone, not the stone according to the jeweller." (Sunil Agarwal, Rishikesh, 2010)* Holistic approaches perfectly embed the patient to support and hold without changing them substantially. The treatments offer a safe space and introduce changes in the environment when necessary. Nutrition and lifestyle (*ahara/vihara*) are crucial parts of the path to recovery.

Unlike western psychological approaches, which focus merely on the mind, healing is impossible if nutrition and lifestyle are not adequate for the patient's inner needs. Considering factors like environment, social and intimate relations, nutrition, exercise, self-care, seasons, weather, health, age and so forth while using this knowledge of the change, transformation and adaption are essential tools for the patient to discover and rediscover connection.

During treatment, positive feelings like safety, tenderness, care, receptive touch, pain reduction, etc., are most likely to convince the patient being on the right path of their experience in connection, recovery and healing.

Society of Friends', Berlin, Research: The stages of traumatic injuries and PTSD translated into ayurveda concepts of the three *doshas*, *ama* and the *gunas*—

Research on the treatment of traumatic injuries, resilience and recovery

At Society of Friends, Berlin, data was collected from treatment options through the unlimited compliance of their patients. They were helpful and supportive for the study after they experienced a reduction of their symptoms of PTSD or when they were able to tackle their drug addiction or sleeplessness. As healing is a complex multifactorial event, Society of Friends, Berlin, focused on increasing resilience, recovery and stable self-care moments.

Key Factors for Resilience and Recovery

According to our findings during the experimental beginning years, the recovery and emotional survival after a traumatic injury or series of them seem to be relying on several key factors:

- previous traumatic experiences
- previous positive experiences of family bonds, care, support, financial security, health
- the individual's stamina (age, health, chronic illnesses, etc.)
- negative co-factors during the event of trauma (eye-witness of other people being traumatised, helper, long term duration of trauma, options to escape or not, kept hostage, weapons, options for self-defence, helplessness)
- positive after-care
- negative after-care
- psychological help provided
- financial situation—support, stable, unstable
- physical damage
- financial damage through or as a result of the traumatising event
- loss of relatives, friends, community
- positive family support
- safe place restored

If the person was alone during the event, they experienced the situation differently than protecting minors, friends or relatives during the traumatic event, attack or threat.

After distress: being in sheltered surroundings, preferably with understanding support, is a better starting position for recovery than experiencing illness, injury, disability or being financially insecure before, during or after the traumatic injury took place.

A key factor on the narrow road of recovery from PTSD, a life in constant distress, seems to be the restauration of the feeling of safety and a compassionate after-care. The ongoing remembrance of the event like it is practiced in psychotherapy, particularly in trauma-psychotherapy groups, definitely plays a crucial role in *not* getting out of traumatic memory.

Some victims reported that they stopped the previous psychotherapy because they needed a "time-out" from the devastating memories recall in the settings. Group therapy seems to be a risk factor for arousal and possibly even generating additional new memories of the event. A survivor of the Berlin Christmas Market Attack in 2016 stated: *During the group sessions, we were exposed to more details that we as individuals had not noticed.*

Hit by falling construction panels, she could not remember how she found herself in a different spot when she tried to get up. During group sittings, the shared stories of other survivors added more horror to her memory. "In the end," she said, "it was hard to find out which one is your memory."

New research has been provided to understand memory and even create false memories. Julia Shaw writes in her book The Memory Illusion: Remembering, Forgetting and the Science of False Memory, pretty similar to the trauma therapist Levine that most people believe that trauma memories are special. She also mentions the self-contradictory situation that on one hand the memories can get suppressed on the other hand the victim is haunted by nightmares and flashbacks.

Therapists and scientists have to rethink treating patients with PTSD by understanding the neuroscience of memories and how memories are created and stored. By grasping the function of memory, ideally, the victim can release and rewrite their memory, focusing on the here and now.

The Key to the Lock of Memory Data

Personal individual memory is never a replica of the event. It adapts to the victim's personality, dealing with the impact and emotions during and after the event. It is important to note that these explanations are not questioning the victim and their credibility. Whatever the victim report are what they genuinely remember—however, it might not be what happened.

Not to be mistaken as an excuse to mistrust the victim of rape, assaults or other terror. It is about creating false memories and not about denying the memory. Confusing the victim with manipulating questions after a traumatic event can lead to wrong assumptions and even implant false memories.

Julia Shaw developed precise guidelines on how to ask the victim about the memory without manipulation. Asking questions about some details might be highly manipulative at the police station or even in court as two people's memory already differ as attention, previous experience, age, position during the event etc. are altered.

Therefore, the question arose in my thoughts: Is there any another way to recover from trauma and PTSD besides repetitive narrative talking of the event? In the daily therapeutic practice, the patients we saw were diligently learning to overcome the horrifying memories.

Could ayurveda and yoga be ways out of the memory trap? Could they possibly create a new pattern to deal with future upsetting and stressful events by meaning-making, structuring life and providing techniques to calm the mind and settle emotions?

Ayurveda: Discovering the Individual Symptoms of the Patient

To provide optimised and precise treatment, multi-dimensional diagnosis is essential. At Society of Friends, Berlin, ayurvedic diagnosis systems and additional detailed biomedical laboratory exams with a close network with biomedical physicians were used. Laboratories and previous medical records, a minimum of the last 5 years, together with a holistic view of emotional influences, understanding of the patient's diet and lifestyle, personal needs and abilities and narratives, created the foundation of a complex and detailed examination.

Measuring Blood pressure, pulse frequency and ordering X-rays were standard to study the overlapping findings of ayurveda and biomedical medicine to give maximum security to the patient. Jumping to conclusions from one single symptom is always wrong. As western diagnosis simplifies various symptoms to one diagnosis (like PTSD), ayurveda provides a detailed symptomatic diagnosis from different observation points.

Therefore, the patients get treated according to their displayed symptoms and the disbalance of doshas and dhatus, blockage of Srotas, aggravation of the gunas and a diagnosis covering a range of possible symptoms and causes. Discovering the patient's symptoms to tailor the treatment is explicitly one of the strengths of ayurveda.

This chapter displays the research done at Society of Friends, Berlin, on traumatised patients according to their displayed symptoms of suffering, pain, avoidance and so on. The symptoms are categorised according to classical ayurvedic diagnosis patterns to develop a tool for treating patients more efficiently and avoiding misleading treatment approaches.

The Society of Friends, Berlin, research led to the following guidelines approved in hundreds of treatments over 40 years. The categories are the results of intense studies with trial and error learning by doing:

An approach from Society of Friends, Berlin, to categorise stages of traumatic injuries and PTSD translated into ayurveda concepts of the three *doshas*, *ama* and the *gunas*

Creating a more efficient way to understand patients with a possible traumatic history, the following guidelines represent the research of the last forty years at Society of Friends, Berlin. There is no other known source to describe the same or a similar structure. Its purpose is to be used and proven by other therapists.

Victims of Trauma might be living for days, years or a lifetime in the first stage of PTS or PTSD, depending on their previous experiences, the setting, the situation and how quickly a safe space has been restored. Depending on the particular trauma and other unknown factors, some patients, including those with dominance in *doshas*, might enter the second stage: tight rope. The first two stages are mostly when the person reaches out for treatment as the effects of the trauma interfere with life. The third stage is more comfortable, as the patient does not reflect on trauma or unpleasant emotions.

However, the experienced numbness or detachment often brings relatives, friends or partners into play who force the patients to seek help. However, the fourth stage is where we usually do not see the patients anymore in the clinic. The decompensation of mental coping mechanisms has led to changes in the personality that might not be reversible. The stage pattern follows the western terms according to P. Levine's trauma stages and translates them into ayurvedic diagnostic language.

Stage 1: Fight of Flight
Vata-Pitta
Stage 2: Tight Rope, High Tension,
Pitta-Vata
Stage 3: Dissociation and Denial,
Kapha
Stage 4: Helplessness and Immobility,
Kapha—Tamas

All the stages do not fall under entirely fixed parameters, but fluid lines within the mind and reaction of the victim oscillate. Nothing in life is a fixed state. Everything that is alive circulates and spirals in transition.

The same is true for the *doshas* and *gunas*. They represent ayurveda as the science of "which" what ends. "We all are constantly changing our inner landscape according to the *doshas* flow," says Prof. Ram Manohar.

These stages represent only experiences based on ideas and ideas based on experiences as work tools from the clinic Society of Friends, Berlin. They need more testing by other therapists until they make a final definition. However, the clear structure helps to establish guidelines of treatment.

Stage 1: The *Vata*-Dominated Fight or Flight Mode

During the traumatising event, a decision has to be made quick:
Can I fight the situation or do I have to escape?
Conditions like prolonged exposure, the overwhelming power of the aggressor or the victim's environment (natural disasters, war, domestic violence, etc.) can prevent the victim from escaping. The victim might remain in stage one or move to stage two, where the dominating emotion is aggressive and self-defensive.

In the clinical practice of Society of Friends, Berlin, primarily patients with stages one and two were seen.

In stage one, the victim tries to figure out the danger ahead. There is no focus on thoughts, actions, etc., because the alert system reaches out in all directions. The mind is shattered and scattered. Concentration, learning and remembering are impaired. The breathing is shallow; the heartbeat rates can rise or drop quickly. Sleeping is difficult due to the high alertness of sensual activity. Mental rest or meditation are not achievable as long as the patient constantly feels like being on the run. A broken continuity of life's essential factors is one of the dominating signs.

Many projects, including healing, are started—but interrupted, left too early and a new project will be around the corner. The financial situation is often disastrous, as attaining regular work is a problem. Nothing gets finished. Loneliness, distrust and lack of faith characterise the patient. Unsteadiness and broken promises let other people avoid the trauma patient in a *Vata*-state.

Stage 2: The Tight Rope or High-Tension Phase of *Pitta-Vata*

Stage two is *pitta*-dominating, yet *Vata* can be present or increased.

Stage two is hypertension state, characterised like a tight rope feeling that is pulled firmly from both sides. Mind and body are in a constant hyper-alert state of self-defence. The person appears often opinionated, self-righteous, overly morale and self-justified or under distress and not paying fully attention to other people's needs. The patients seem to be unable to pay respect or give space to others or take criticism. A classic question could be: "Don't you know who I am?"

Narcissistic traits can isolate them even from their loved ones and perpetuate more traumatic content in the family. The trauma content that is hidden deep inside the personality can lead to domestic violence, offensive sexual behaviour or physical abusive dominant behaviour as much as it can open doors to careers.

Aggressive behaviour, intolerance, irritability and impatience often lead to short-tempered outbursts that end relationships that could have been meaning-making. It has to be interpreted as fear, vulnerability and usually low self-esteem, but there is no time or insight to reach out for help and the person feels victimised. A facade of being "tough" constructs around them.

The patients seek help primarily because of their sleeplessness, drug abuse of recreational drugs like cocaine, speed, Ritalin, often combined with a "downer" like alcohol, Benzodiazepine, Marijuana or pain killers. Persisting tension in the body occurs that no pain killer or massage might relieve. The patients often show signs of hyperactivity, restlessness and tend to participate in risky behaviour like risky sports, risky sexual practices or dangerous driving.

At Society of Friends, Berlin, an increased number of reoccurring and often complicated physical injuries were seen in these individuals, as they mentioned: "I thought I am indestructible," *Patient D., 2019.*

They are on a dangerous and edgy path, just as tense as walking on a tight rope. The victim's only option to deal with the traumatic experience seems to be by fighting it constantly. Symptoms like sleeplessness and overdosing on barbiturates (downers) or upper drugs (cocaine, Ritalin, speed) deny the body's pleas for proper rest, resulting in exhaustion and the feeling of losing power and control. The feeling of loss of power and control could lead to spontaneous decisions to commit suicide. Therefore, stimulating treatments should be avoided, even though the patient might complain about the lack of power and the increasing exhaustion.

The victim might move onto stage three if they cannot find proper treatment and rest.

Stage 3: The Dissociation and Denial—*Kapha* Dominated

This stage is reigned by *Kapha Dosha* and can show signs of worsening through the psychological quality of *tamas*. This stage can be interpreted as burn-out as a modern and widely accepted description, perfectly explaining it as a phase after the pitta or fiery phase.

Stage three is characterised by dissociation and denial. The body feels numb and physical activity is often challenging because of mental inhibition or physical exhaustion.

Pleasure avoidance is another typical mental expression. Victims often report not allowing themselves to perform sports or any joyful activity like participating in dance or social activities. They often suffer from compulsive behaviour disorders that do not let them leave the house.

Financial problems often increase and become threatening to health and social living. The patients do not open their mailbox, answer emails and do not pay bills—their health decreases due to a lack of interest in any physical activity. Lack of spiritual belief, hope and loss of meaning are critical emotional responses and could even lead to life-threatening behaviour.

A person who has lost contact and hope has lost meaning in life. Life turns into a vegetative process, where security and isolation is the primary goal. The absence of global meaning leaves the patient in an insecure mental state, where they feel surrounded by optional threats. These threats can become highly toxic as they often result from a false meaning (vaccination introduces microchips in the body, a virus is genetically produced to destroy the world and more).

For some people, the anxious preoccupation with the event is an attempt to find meaning in it. This trial to meaning is the deep hope to gain control over future events. It is the hope to arrive at a cognitive resolution that would allow the victim to integrate the event and, therefore, can move away from it.

It is vital to carefully introduce valid meaning-making through positive physical and emotional experiences instead. The body as a safe place, not as a place that gets invaded by its irrational responses. Focusing on negative meanings like conspiracy theories or other fearful content will continue in reproducing unreasonable fears.

Stage 4: Helplessness and Immobility: *Kapha* and *Tamas*

If the patient has not received proper psychological or psychiatric intervention or other care and possible lifestyle changes, food, nutrition and social environment, they might be experiencing stage four, characterised by hopelessness and helplessness. Patients with these traits are usually not seen by complementary medicine practitioners, simply as they do not leave the house and have given up on any changes.

Symptoms occurring with signs of amnesia can make communication difficult. Other symptoms include constant tiredness (fatigue), lack of concentration and willpower, lack of interest and social activities, physical inactivity or hoarding. The victim is living a self-isolated life in despair. Patients and relatives express this as "a feeling of being dead while being alive." Some of them end up homeless. Social and financial dilapidation become primarily unavoidable.

An inadequate diet reflects a lack of understanding and self-care. Unfortunately, it also reflects unsupportive life circumstances that do not allow or guarantee proper nutrition. Patients surviving natural disasters, escaping war or financially disastrous situations or unstable living conditions often do not have access to clean water, decent healthy food and enough sleep. Healthy food can be pricy and some people have not been able to get the proper education to make sensible food choices or learn how to prepare suitable food one has to consider this when treating patients with diverse backgrounds.

The option of choice is a luxury for most people. Fast food consumption is quick and easy but creates *Ama* and supports inflammatory processes in the body and the brain. Inflammatory destruction in the brain, poor food choices, slow digestion and lack of mobility contribute to depression.

Classification and Description of the Stages in Trauma Experience

Not all the above changes of the personality and not all possible alterations described for each stage might occur in the traumatised individual. The way life takes the patient is not necessarily from 1 to 4. It is not an inevitable way towards the worst and hopeless state.

Sometimes, only a few behavioural changes seen after the intervention can start making a significant difference to the perspective; some changes and adaptions can be hidden on purpose or unconsciously and even an experienced therapist might have difficulties noticing them instantly. Sometimes the person is not even aware of being traumatised, as they have never experienced anything different. Sometimes there can be additional symptoms.

The above layout of stages is merely a clinical experienced working tool to help practitioners dealing more efficiently and compassionately with traumatised patients. The diagnose "trauma" or "PTSD" classifies a wide range of emotional and physical changes and disorders. Therefore, it is important to have handy solutions and classifications for treatment that could meet the individual's demand and their particular and unique history.

Additional to the ayurvedic diagnosis and treatment, yoga therapy offers practical guidelines. *Pranayama,* for instance, turned out to be an effective tool in my practice to modify stress-related patterns, like anxiety, panic or sleeplessness as erratic breathing patterns, often unknown to the patient, are important in diagnosing and treating PTSD.

Another example could be the development of Compulsive Behaviour Disorder. The extreme urge to control is so well established in the person's daily routine that the patient often does not notice the source of it. They often think that it's just a "habit." These "shrugs" in fact consume enormous amounts of energy and are actually creating more distress or even isolation instead of the desired connection. Organising life and trying to control as much as possible leads to disintegration of the self with the needed adaptive flow.

More often, we can observe messiness and hoarding, which basically come from the same root of trying to hold on and control. Trauma can leave the victim with a heightened vulnerability in some cases; however, we can also see the opposite. Neither of this is an indicator whether the trauma had happened or not or if the victim is trying to step out of the-even often unknown—experience.

The person with heightened vulnerability might even have a better position by being aware of difficulties and might seek for help, while a person who is not able to admit vulnerability can act out in an abusive and narcissistic way. Without insight and/or treatment, both adaptions to trauma have a high chance to pass on the trauma to the next generations. Society declares adaptions as a normal behaviour and even rewards aggressive and manipulative ways with leading positions in economy and politics, while the hyperreactive person often finds salvation in care taking positions and self-exploitation.

So, where to start a treatment? Cognitive treatments take years in not only getting a space with a therapist, as we discussed earlier, but the question remains, does an insight really change the adaption?

Many patients came to me, saying: "I knew before where it all came from and there is stuff I just don 't want to speak about"—the resistance to speak about certain events is often interpreted as a lack of compliance, that the patient resists a change.

From a compassionate perspective we instead would argue that the resistance can be a shelter in order not to be overwhelmed by the content of the memory— and by its often irrational content. As we have seen earlier that the memory of traumatic events is not a clear and precise picture of the event therefore it gets changed by each questioning, manipulation or emotional attachments. More important is the fact that the rationalising mind does not deliver healing per se.

What can ayurveda provide instead?

Gut Brain, Heart Brain and Skin Brain. Apart from the brain, ayurveda considers the heart, gut and also skin as centres where the mind is very active. Therefore, the gut, heart and skin can influence the mind. Ayurveda uses this principle to influence the mind through specific treatments. (Manohar, 2019, transcript from a lecture.)

It was observed patients with a background of addiction (mostly *Pitta*) seem to be more likely to accept and integrate new routines and rituals than those patients who had fallen out of any daily routine (*Tamas, Kapha*).

Table: An Overview of the Research on Hundreds of Patients at Society of Friends, Berlin in the Years 1997-2020.

Neurological Changes	Physiological Changes	Psychological Changes
hyperactivity, hyper-reactive, easily startled	increased pulse rate, irritable	extreme emotions, hypersensitivity, easily startled into fear and anxiety of things that could happen, fear of diseases or future disasters, end of the world scenarios.
hallucinations	sweating	nightmares
disturbance of vision, lightheadedness, dizziness under stressful situations, fainting	difficulties breathing, shallow, pausing, paradox, irregular breathing	sudden mood swings from anxiety to anger. Fear to aggressiveness.
vertigo	cold sweat, cold hands, cold feet as well as sudden heat flushes (if *Pitta* is higher)	low self—esteem, low self—worth often in paradox combination with narcissism
tremors, trembling, shaking	tension and dysfunctional muscles, mostly neck, back, shoulders	fear, phobia, feeling of being outside of one's own body, dissociation of body parts
problems to find words, expressing oneself	late bedtimes, early awakening, too little rest	avoidance of people, places, smells and other common triggers
forgetfulness, cannot focus	asthma, feeling of not breathing enough air in	psychiatric drugs
disturbances of the memory of the event (s)	skin diseases	overdosing medications, alcohol, recreational drug abuse of downing drugs

	pre-menstrual syndrome	fear of the future
	low or hyper—interest in sexual activity	loss of trust
	immunity problems through high cortisol levels: prone to infections or not getting ill at all, cancer disposition at higher risk	self—hate, neglecting one's own needs
		self-harming behaviour like cutting, bulimia, anorexia, overeating, binge eating, feeling of having a knot in the stomach
		restlessness

Second Stage: High Tension Pitta—Vata

Neurological Changes	Physiological Changes	Psychological Changes
mental: tunnel-like concentration, no creative side thinking	shortened shallow breathing, paradox breathing	over—reaction to everyday situations: overly aggressive, opinionated, compulsive, even violent and destructive
no multitasking, hectic	aggressive mouth-breathing	hyperactivity, restlessness, overworking
bad memory	disturbed digestion, hyperacidity, ulcers. cannot tolerate longer times without food, unstable blood sugar	uncontrolled use of recreational drugs, alcohol, painkillers, sleepers, abuse of prescribed drugs

only short-term attention possible	high blood pressure, high blood pressure episodes	risky sexual behaviour
addiction-prone	skin problems, reddishness of the face, neck, sweaty	risky behaviour: sports, driving
anger, impatience	overheated body, intolerant to higher temperature	self-destructive behaviour: anorexia, bulimia, cutting
high-stress response	tendency to inflammations, herpes, skin rashes	abusive behaviour
high cortisol levels	injuries	regular use of recreational drugs, overdosing in particular with cocaine, heroin, speed, crystal meth, etc
use of limited areas of the brain, major use of amygdala	restless legs syndrome, "everything is geared up for tension"	overuse of sleepers and benzodiazepine
	enlarged pupils	panic attacks, manic behaviour, fear of being poisoned or cursed
	sour sweat, sweaty palms, feet, inguinal region	demonstration of power, narcissistic
		hypersensitivity to smells, sounds, events as a remain of high *Vata*

Stages 3 and 4: Dissociation and Denial: *Kapha, Tamas and* Possible Depletion of *Ojas**

Neurological Changes	Physiological changes	Psychological Changes
loss of memory of past events unable to deal with daily activities	disturbance of hormonal balance, thyroid problems like hypo-activity or Hashimoto thyroiditis, glucose imbalances, insulin intolerance	denial of the trauma inability to get motivated resisting all changes, loss of hope
interruption/loss of the memory of the traumatic event	low physical motivation, sluggishness, no sexual desire, no appetite	depending on others, dirty appearance, not looking after oneself
reliving the traumatic event, flashbacks, no reality	cannot start or finish activities as overwhelmed by exhaustion, sweat, short breath	inability to accomplish intellectual goals, loss of perspective and purpose in life
nightmares, daydreaming of horror events, threatening and abuse	large stools, oily stools, slow digestion, smelly, weight gain or severe weight loss, depending on caretakers	constant feeling of danger or not feeling anything at all
interruption of the emotional memory and the feelings of the traumatising event, numbness, dissociation	shallow breathing, paradox breathing	loss of spirituality and belief
drug abuse, addiction	increase of BP amplitude	depression and inappropriate behaviour, defensive

sleep disorder, often too much sleeping, drowsy	very high pulse—rate and low blood pressure, high blood pressure with low amplitude, very cold hands, feet and back, cold sweat, sticky sweat, sweaty back and palms, cold skin	messy life, hoarding

The sacred way of healing in Indian tradition has many faces. On one of my journeys to the sacred places of the Ganga, there was a patient who suffered from massive sexual and physical trauma and previous traumatic loss of all family members. The priest (*pandit*) we visited went into the mountains for ten days to deal with all spiritual entities that he discovered in their case and then invited her to do offerings to all the members by naming, giving presents and then letting them go.

It was an incredible process to observe. There was a gathering in Haridwar (Uttarakhand, India) on an auspicious day. All people who suffered from the loss of family members were seated with their respected priests and astrologists, carrying photos and belongings, food and sandalwood, ghee and rice to perform the ritual. The sheer presence of hundreds of people united in their feeling of grief was overwhelming.

Grief, sadness and mourning are not welcome in western societies' modern hectic life. Loss seems is for losers. It appears that there is no time to stop the daily business—and realise, feel the emptiness that a loss leaves behind. The loss of connection is painful but needs to be experienced in order to grow out of it.

Encountering unpleasant emotions and integrating them into the personal narrative is valuable. Ayurveda allows the patient to go beyond the grief and mourn by connecting these feelings to the life's story. With non-verbal experiences like wellness, soothing, comfort and care, patients can allow themselves to dive deeper into their original self.

How to transfer ancient holistic ayurvedic treatments into a western medical practice location?

Understanding the importance of rituals and routines like *ahara-vihara* (lifestyle and nutrition) as key tools of ayurveda to restore a person's balance is essential to achieve the best results in treatment. However, copying Indian rituals and manners is not a solution, as patients need to find authenticity not cultural appropriation in practice and treatment. Understanding one's own cultural and family roots and upbringing is important to establish a healthy self-identity.

Each society develops its codes of understanding, support, integrity, rituals and routines. Ayurveda emphasises living according to one's own authentic needs and respecting others. However, we might not be able to translate the western perspective on meaning in life, which is a key moment in my eyes for recovery. We need to see that the concepts of eastern traditions differ. I think this is one of the problems if a different cultural background is used to cover up deficiencies. Toxic positivity can be seen as a result of the attempt to find meaning in another philosophy, not in oneself.

The meaning is often described as a "thing", according to Voss, which means it is something material and less an experience or an inner call. Eva Illiouz writes about love in times of capitalism from the same perspective that the role models that society imposes on us decide over meaning and happiness versus status and materialism.

By copying parts out of socio-cultural context from another complex society and their spiritual, religious and other meaning, we would not be able to meet the patient's individual needs. We could even increase feelings of being alienated in a fake social surrounding. Chanting names of Indian deities, changing one's own name into some foreign language, using the prefix goddess, wearing exotic clothes and turbans might serve the narcissistic—self of many traumatised people—but is not a required prop for a therapeutic healer in ayurveda or yoga—

These new identities are a misunderstanding as role model for treatment. As C.G. Jung had expressed this clearly in his famous commentary on the "Secret of the Golden Flower," an ancient Taoist text. *"Es ist dem westlichen Menschen aufgegeben, das Östliche anzuempfinden"—It is the westerners ability to close-by-feel the eastern mind* (vague translation by the author as the original precise words cannot be accurately translated, only interpreted).

Feeling close to something does not mean integrating it into one's own beliefs and meaning. Meaning-making in the west 21st century is not the same as in ancient India; however, emotions and primary needs are the same.

Under the right circumstances with the right intention, it is possible to transfer emotional knowledge and meaning into a patient's life without alienating the patient from her own culture. Ayurveda and yoga introduce patients carefully through their individual experiences to an underlying common sense of meaning-making. They encourage meaning-making by experiencing a safe place and contentment.

Ayurveda and Yoga science describe the proper use of all the necessary tools to define and treat the shattered mind and the body.

The Triune Brain—An Inquiry into Recent Neuroscience to Answer Questions about how ayurveda Works

Question 1: Am I safe?

Neuroscience differentiates behavioural patterns from the reptilian part of the brain—the brain stem, the instinctually fastest response to distress, hunger and mating. It primarily deals with the question:

Am I safe?

Manas is defined as a part of consciousness in the lower sensory mind. Manas is a bit similar to a storage, it takes information in only. Manas does not create a context, nor gives meaning or evaluates. It is a primarily the instinct based part of the consciousness. Information is collected but they are not naturally leading to evolving in consciousness or skills.

Manas represents the faculty to store only. As we know this ability can be reduced, altered, compromised but diseases like Parkinson, Alzheimer's, etc., where in the beginning the recording of new memory content only is vanishing, but long-term memory is active. The manas aspect is actively checking the environment and stores this information. For a traumatised patient, the manas are often partially "deactivated", so only a few information is stored. This means the patient's ability to receive information about safety is only active which leads to high responsiveness without the judgment of the other faculties of the mind.

Question 2: Am I loved?

The limbic parts of the brain are working on emotions and feelings and develop later in human life. The question asked could be: Am I loved? It involves social behaviour as well as self-identity. Citta is connected to the storage manas by moving the content like the ocean in a stream of thoughts. To stop this stream of thoughts, the ripples of the constantly ongoing inner discussion, is the aim of yoga.

As Patanjali can be quoted: yoga aims to stop the moving of the consciousness. Its inconsistency, however, is deeply connected to our identity.

As the identity is experienced through reflection of others, it is not as solid as we think.

In ayurveda, the foundation of self—identity is a basket in the three doshas as in Prkrt; however, it needs the interaction with food, the surrounding and all the influences to unfold. Only the connection to all the influences in life brings the Dosha Prkrt into action, in a healthy way of benevolence or in a way of illness and conflict.

The Citta is, according to some authors, outside of our awareness, what modern psychology would call: *the unconscious*. However, according to ayurveda, there is nothing like *the Unconscious*. We have to remember how recently the idea of the Unconscious just evolved in the west and it is not a thing, there is no material proof. It is a concept of an idea as much as we see concepts of ideas in any other medical, traditional medical or even shamanic context.

We should not forget this that the concepts we use in the western world are not written in stone. But more we should be stunned by the precise description of different aspects of consciousness, emotional aspects, feelings, memory and the aspects of insanity given in the classic texts of ayurveda and yoga and being close to the latest neuroscientific research.

One part of the Citta is acting in union with *manas* and collecting data. When Mansa can remember the room, it is Citta that remembers how he felt in the room or what was astonishing, frightening, interesting. And keep on going over it again and again when we weren't sure about the situation. Or when we felt aroused, agitated, disturbed, uncontrolled, fearful, etc.

The other part of Citta is more of a filter and can be actively used. While we cannot filter out our general sensory input, we can learn how to modify our reaction and even silence it.

Discovering the Citta is the unfortunate moment in meditation. Instead of enjoying the quietness of a non—moving body and nothing to do, the Citta starts to get agitated and plays all kinds of past experiences, questions, insecurities, unsolved problems or making even problems out nothing. Some authors, like in Yoga and Psychotherapy, Desikachar, describe the situation in a clear picture: as if nothing is life on broadcast, the Citta replays and old movies are seen, as if all memory traces and impressions from the past begin to flash on the screen, wavering and repetitive.

Ayurveda and Yoga can unfold their ability to restructure memories and modify the response to past experiences on the screen of their presence.

Question 3: Who Am I?

The Information from the evolutionary later developed frontal lobe parts connected to problem solving, memory, behaviour, personality enable the person to ask: Who am I? What did I learn from it? Thus, reflecting the most abstract form of thinking and self-inquiry. We are all familiar with the steps that the children take when they move from their mumbling to naming their caretakers to finally discovering the power of the "I".

We also know that apes and crows can identify the "I" and even do have a clear image of themselves and can differentiate themselves from other beings. They identify themselves in the mirror. We see random brain injuries leading to the loss of the image of the self.

In ayurveda and yoga, the Shamkhya philosophy describes the Ahamkara, the "I" maker or ego—creator, clearly as an important factor in the evolution of the consciousness (Aham: I—ness, Kara—making). Basically meaning in owning one's narrative, one can learn from the past. This is only possible if a strong sense of "I" is existing.

In trauma, the "I" function of the self-making can be harmed so badly that personality disorders can evolve. The discussion here is about Borderline Personality, where the self is trying to find hold by adapting to other people's traits and styles.

The immense fear of abandonment is vital, as the personality loses its mirroring identification with the other (there is more to say, but I wanted to name one example). Young children can show symptoms after traumatising events of excessive anger, as they are not capable of containing the emotions in a stable self. They are over-personalising. Constant gaslighting by narcissistic parents can lead to self-doubt and questioning one's owns emotions and perceptions. This leaves a person vulnerable to future abuse in narcissistic relationships.

The next question would arise what love can look like in a person with a healthy sense of self and "I" and what can be mistaken for love in a weakened self.

The end of the comparison list between the Triune brain and the ayurveda/yoga Philosophy matches is *Buddhi*. Buddhi evolves in stages. Each stage is characterised by experience, reflection, self-reflection. It is an evolution in a healthy "I"-ness.

While the previous faculties of the mind or consciousness are instinct driven, Buddhi marks the change into a different cause of action. The person is now able to make decisions that even might be in contradiction to its instinctual impulse. Even past experiences can be questioned, as Buddhi clearly acts from the healthy source of the being.

We can name Buddhi the pacemaker of our therapeutic interventions and of the person's general ability to heal by right and intelligent decision making. *Buddhi* can decide and leave the old route by choice. Its development and training through awareness, sensual positive experiences and breath control can change the traumatised patient. *Buddhi* is the faculty to discriminate and eradicate what is not necessary. *Buddhi* provides meaning-making by concentrating on fruitful and creative solutions. It provides choices.

Developing the ability to make active choices, even as potential, is the focus of direction for Trauma Therapy. It induces hope and defines how treatment guidelines are present. Using ayurveda and yoga techniques and bringing them into a sincere practice can make change happen. It is said that: "Nothing changes if nothing changes.". Change is described as the potential, willingness, ability and diligent regime necessary to turn the potential into a real-life changer that lasts.

Buddhi, by definition, has a decision-making function. It can decide to permit some memories and not others (the author's change of perception of unpleasant touch to pleasant touch, the idea of a safe space). Buddhi maintaining detachment and observation towards memory traces can allow those to pass away and dissipate.

These recent discoveries of the brain parts and their particular functions in the sense of self-identity, decision-making and meaning-making have been made with extensive studies worldwide. Brain scans and computer tomography and the descriptions from Charaka are merely empiric studies through observation, self-inquiry and awareness.

In neurological function, humans can monitor and observe their behaviour, decision-making and even their brain by observing how tasks get done and problems get solved, etc. They can modify their response to alterations in their life by learning.

Traumatised patients, therefore, can enable to control and modify their distress response through continuous learning and re-learning. Repetition and consistency are the tools for rewiring the distress response. Yoga and ayurveda deliver a rich history of detailed and various techniques. These techniques vary from relaxing to invigorating, from hyperventilation to breath-hold, warmth and pampering to freeze and pain. They are part of a complex concept to select and administer the correct treatment.

The Triune Brain has overlapping discoveries with the concepts of the creation of consciousness according to Samkhya philosophy and, on a medical level, with Charaka's empirical observation.

The Eastern Patient and The Western Patient

Without compliance, all effort is useless and in vain. Traumatised patients, despite having a solid motivation in general to change their faith and either *"go back to normal. To the time before"* or start *"living their lives"* ("So far I haven't lived, I did not even age as I kept myself away from all times and life itself," Patient O., 2020).

Patients in India generally do not observe these drastic and rapid changes in emotions during the ayurveda treatments. Most Indian patients are still living steady family relations, with regular daily life rhythms, set aims and regular meals. The standard rule in India is more likely to follow a doctor's advice than in the west. Paying respect to elderly or more experienced people is a pillar in Indian societies (*societies* as a tribute to the many different cultures inside India, yet they do have the respect for the elderly in common).

The eastern patient is less likely to invest money in a project, like seeing a doctor for health and then deciding to sabotage the healing process. Yet this behaviour is, unfortunately, widespread in the west. In particular, traumatised patients more often practice consciously or unconsciously a wide range self-sabotaging behaviour.

Self-sabotage is a massive hindrance in the journey of recovery. However, the discovery of embracing the motherly kindness of the ayurveda treatments and the soothing breathing techniques from yoga made a difference in future compliance. The patient feels encouraged to seriously try again. They start making an effort. If they fall off the wagon, they get support and be up again.

In ayurveda/yoga treatments, punishment, devaluation, humiliation, guilt and shame should be absent. Patients start feeling valued again with care. This new feeling of self-appreciation is soothing and self-care arising, it opens the way to recovery. Unlike psychiatric medicine prescription, the patient can perform self-control with positive feedback and never an adverse judgment. Self-empowering without pressure and expectations, in order of being connected to a meaningful life and appreciation, can change the patient's common assumption that the world is an unpleasant place and one does not deserve any love or care.

After years, many patients come back to confirm that their new openness changed their feeling toward themselves. They discovered they want to be good to themselves and there is no point after being damaged to continue self-sabotage. The way to recovery through self-appreciation and meaning-making through positive feelings and the cultivation of self-care within a system that provides answers is a powerful alternative to medication.

However, other therapy models used supportively are sometimes less needed. Ayurveda and yoga present a richness and diversity of therapy modules within a context that needs to be fully rediscovered and used for the benefit of the patients.

Patanjali and the Wisdom of the Yoga Sutras in the Context of Trauma

This chapter focuses on the inquiry of the mind through breathing and *asanas* as tools for self-observation, endurance, stamina and resilience. As yoga has become so popular in the west, it thrives here for constant authentication through stories and rumours, not, however, in diligent and dedicated practice to self-inquiry.

Self-optimising is often a hindrance on the way to self-knowledge. Self-optimisation does two things: it brings people into a stressful practice as there is always something to achieve and it takes away contentment and happiness. The idea of self-optimisation stops people with lower self-esteem, even from starting. At Society of Friends, Berlin, we have seen many more burn-out patients who had undergone yoga teacher training rather than in any other profession. However, they again reported massive stress as the pattern of low self-esteem, overfilling expectations, etc., continued to havoc on those patients.

115

Yoga Classes, Namaste and Trauma: The Role of Yoga Teaching and Therapy of Trauma in Context

While we can trace back the origins of yoga thousands of years back to the Indian subcontinent, we have to admit that what is now performed not only in the west but flooding back to the east is a broken system. During the British colonialism in India Indians tried to prove the British that Indian culture was rational and healthy and sophisticated, which was already caught in a trap to prove certain aspects of western science in order to be acknowledged.

The Rosenberg Akademie (REAA) in Birstein, Germany, had been an example of a safe space where students of yoga and ayurveda can study in a sheltered environment while pursuing their yoga education and the related Ayurveda Yoga Chikitsa for many decades. The Academy had been free of doctrine towards yogic "styles" and open to all yoga schools and confessions. The staff compromised with experienced teachers who had qualifications as therapists, Heilpraktiker (naturopaths), GPs or psychiatrists.

A trained psychotherapist with a highly profiled background of academic studies on Indology, Prof. Martin Mittwede, offers lifelong guidance in the field. A controlling network of teachers, the head of the academy and office workers, were open to suggestions and complaints. Unfortunately, during the Corona Pandemic, the academy decided to close its doors for further Yoga Teacher educations. Only the remaining Ayurveda Yoga Chikitsa, Ayurveda Yoga therapy classes held by Professor Mittwede and myself are still in practice.

The ayurveda concepts of care and shelter are the pillars in which the yoga training in the west and elsewhere can unfold safely. However, we are always alert to rumours of sexual assault through therapists and teachers all over the world.

"Mind is derived from the Trigunas following the Samkhya System of thought. Ayurveda explains that the mind is derived from the Trigunas. Rajas and Tamas are considered as the faults of the human mind. The goal is to tame Rajas and Tamas and bring it within the dominance of Sattva."(Vaidya Manohar, private discussion in Birstein, 2019)

"The moon in the lake is not the reflection of the self, as the moon itself is only the reflection of the sun." (Ram Manohar, Birstein, private discussion, 2019)

The Yoga Sutras

The Yoga Sutras are nowadays a standard of yoga education in the west. However, their deep essence is often not understood, yoga in western countries is often dominated by falsifications and trivialisations of inner spiritual experiences and by focussing on physical exercise. For therapy purposes, the *Sutras* are a milestone in understanding the function of the mind and therefore influencing patterns of behaviour.

The *Yoga Sutra* is one of the oldest texts books on yoga available today to the English-speaking public and has been translated into hundreds of languages. Other ancient scriptures are *Gheranda Samhita, Hatha Yoga Pradipika, Shiva Samhita. The Bhagavad Gita,* part of the vast historical epos *Mahabharata*, is also a text of yoga. Besides *Patanjali* and the *Gita*, most texts are currently not well translated or the topic of yoga is not as popular as the *Sutras* yet.

The *Sutras* give detailed advice on observing the mind and are no guidelines for physical practice. The only position is basically "the seat." However, the Sutras of Patanjali are very complex in their original Sanskrit language. Sanskrit allows and offers a lot of space for interpretations, analysis and speculation. So the language of Sanskrit offers precision as well as it allows interpretation. We truly have no accurate meaning of what Patanjali did or did not say. The Sanskrit that is used for the Yoga Sutras has, according to Nicolas Sutton, no verbs to fill in the gap in meaning. Phrases remain obscure.

The instructions are about the practice of controlling *citta-vrtti*. It is a very systematic course outline from how to start the practice in order to reveal the truth. *Patanjali* is strictly emphasising diligent self-study. Therefore, the Eightfold Path (Ashtanga Yoga, not to be mixed with the yoga style by Pattabhi Jois) should be understood as an instructional text for self-observation and self-practice. The different chapters deal with the inquiry into the nature of the mind.

The mind is described in all its faculties, the functions of each aspect within the framework of the I, *ahamkara* and how each aspect connects to other aspects. How to control the function of the mind through yoga is the scientific approach that Patanjali has laid out as a path to liberation.

Is not all Yoga "Therapy" by its very nature?

"There is no coming to consciousness without pain. People will do anything, no matter how absurd, in order to avoid facing their own soul. One does not become enlightened by imagining figures of light, but by making the darkness conscious." C.G. Jung, own translation by the author

Is not all yoga therapy in its very meaning of healing as it brings light into the dark corners of the self? It is and it is not. Yoga therapy for treating trauma, distress, anxiety or a broken shoulder, chronic pain syndrome, slip disc, etc., is not an aim for the liberation of the self. The goal can be much smaller than self-liberation. It can be a relief from symptoms and a way to control arousals, increase resilience, create a peaceful state of mind and increase stamina and flexibility. Nevertheless, the word "yoga" is used with several techniques from the eightfold path to improve the patient's health and overall well-being.

If *Patanjali* is dealing explicitly with the liberation from the fluctuations of the mind and achieving mental equilibrium and peace, further experienced as *samadhi*—why is there YOGA THERAPY?

Yoga, again, is a word that has undergone a shift in its meaning on its journey to the west. Widely understood in western countries as an exercise regime with diverse spiritual backgrounds, it has become what the yoga teacher Michel Bleier, New York, called "household yoga." Besides discussing what "real yoga" is, it is remarkable how tiny bits of yoga science can change a person's life's perspective, feeling, response, pain reduction, meaning-making, recovery, resilience or even healing on a physical or mental level. The International Association of Yoga Therapists lays possible improvements:

Besides ending, managing or reducing pain and suffering from the cause function will be improved through yoga therapy. Yoga therapy further should be used to move forward to health and wellbeing, change unhealthy conditions and nevertheless empower the people to become their own teachers and healers. The last point of the seven goals is to teach and share to support and inspire other to be as awake, vibrant as possible so that every moment is filled with awe.

This goals from Mark Stephens make me feel uncomfortable as we discussed earlier that toxic positivity like in the expectation of awe in life at every moment sets unrealistic goals and leads to suffering. The victim will feel outside again, left behind in a life that seems to be an ongoing Instagram feed if you just work hard enough on your issues. Or if you wish strong enough. So I would like to distance myself from these goals. How would I define it? As a joined journey into the open sea.

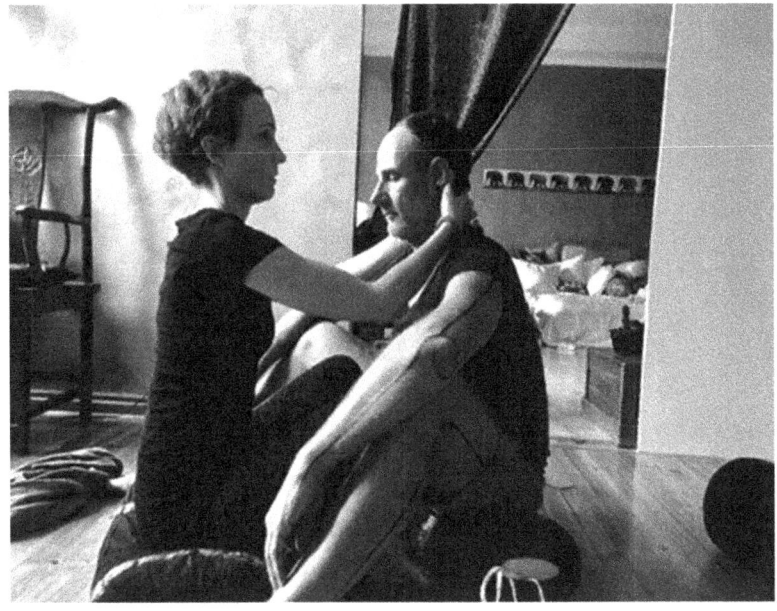

Photo: the author. Two students are exploring the spinal movement in twisted *asanas* during Ayurveda Yoga Teacher Training, 2018

Yoga Therapy uses Patanjali's clear and sophisticated layout to discover the secrets of the mind and yoga therapy uses asana and pranayama practice to overcome illness or restrictions of the physical body, loss of healthy breathing patterns and is helping to find a way into the serenity of meditation, as well as pratyahara or meditation, all according to the ability and preparation of the student.

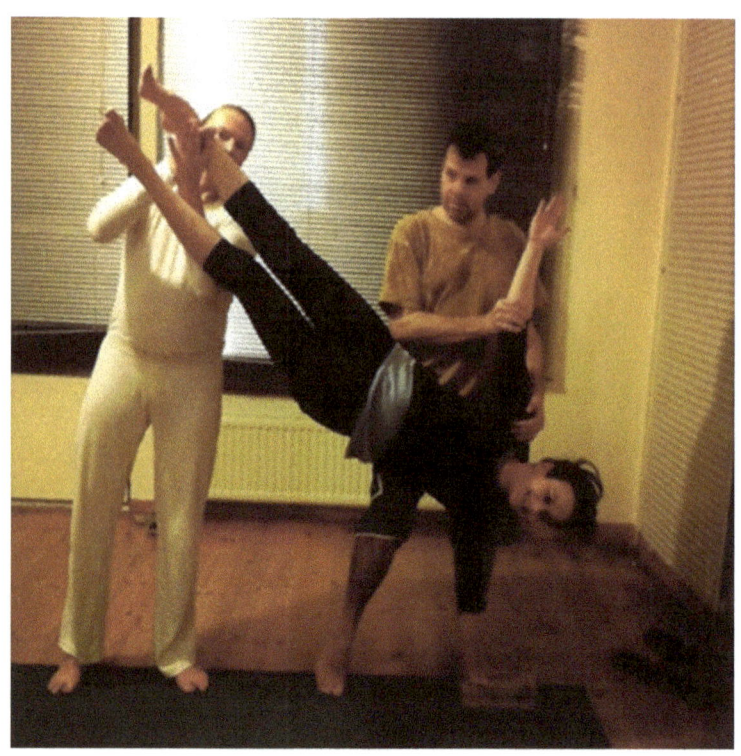

Photo: the author. Students are exploring special techniques to induce a feeling of lightness. Support through their friends is experienced as a safe place, even in a situation that is unknown and even a bit scary. From: yoga group Yolli, 2009

Yoga as well as Therapy unfortunately have become an open playground for interpretations, theories, cultural appropriation, trial or even as a substitute for Therapy in general. Rooted in Patanjali's Yoga Sutras are several schools, like in Mysore, Chennai, India, run by Desikachar, Mohandas, Patabhi Jois and several other teachers. B.K.S. Iyengar in Pune, Usha, and Surinder Singh in Rishikesh and thousands of unnamed teachers developed their own unique styles of treating patients with yoga therapy.

From the west, there is almost every school of yoga and yoga therapy claiming to be rooted in the Yoga Sutra. Often enough we discover an unfortunate mix of interpretations of Christian background beliefs in order to make them more palatable, less radical freedom oriented, for the western student.

Patanjali emphasises that yoga only should be practiced when the student is physically and mentally healthy and at their best. So the term "Yoga Therapy" seems a contradiction in itself at first. Is it justified to adapt the techniques for minor purposes (compared to liberation) like pain control, coping with stress and other symptoms? Or could be these symptoms rooted in the inner quest of "who am I"?

The Yoga Sutras' Empiric Approach Towards Understanding the functions of the so called Mind

Mentioning the Yoga Sutras in an ayurveda context on Trauma I feel is sensible as it fills a gap that I personally find in ayurveda when it comes to psychological or psychiatric disturbances—if we classify those now with a term of western thinking—The gap is the one of a self—analysis of the function of the mind.

As Professor Ram Manohar states*, *There is no ayurvedic psychology, there is only ayurvedic psychiatry.* (Manohar, 2018)

The Yoga Sutras of Patanjali give a proper guideline to discover how the different faculties of the mind works and how to control the movement of thoughts and the linked emotions. The presented Case Studies in Chapter four display emotional disturbances and uncontrolled movement of the mind in the traumatised patient.

In my clinical practice, yoga therapy has been added to the ayurveda treatment plans successfully and supports the goal of a peaceful mind. Through yoga techniques, it was possible to design treatments that allow the patients to continue their work of mental self-regulation.

Discovering self-deceive, patterns of avoidance, pleasure avoidance, the roots of denial, fear and anxiety by simply altering the breathing pattern and/or creating awareness in a pose (*asana*) has been proven a simple and effective method to achieve tranquillity and change in life. Meditation (*dhyana*) and retrieval of the senses (*pratyahara*) in combination with posture (*asana*) and breathing (*pranayama*), are faculties that are of tremendous value in the treatment of trauma/PTSD.

Ayurvedic treatments like abhyanga or shirodhara are all relying on an ayurvedic therapist for application. Yoga therapy, however, can be practiced alone by the patient at any time and when it is needed most. Yoga empowers the patient to actively contribute to the treatment process in recovery or resilience.

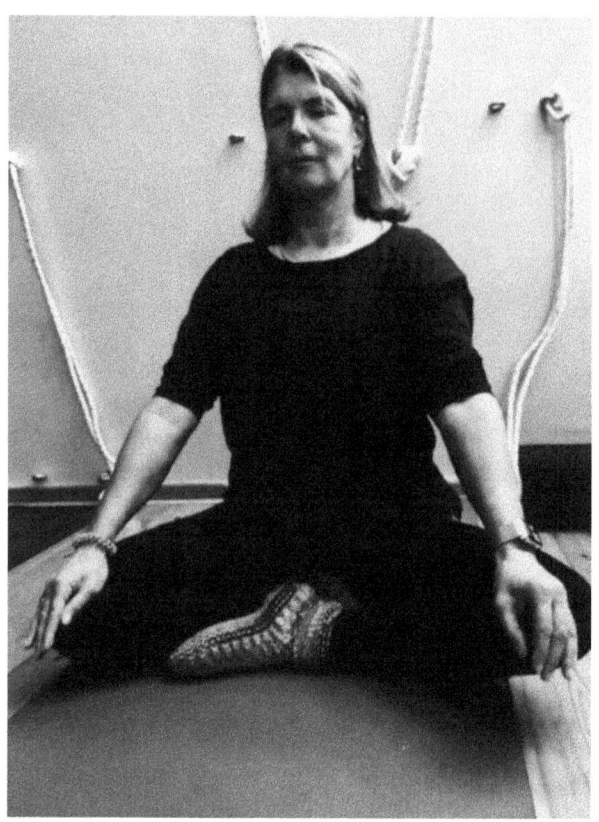

Photo credit: the author, Student M. performing the Swastikasana under direct instructions of her student friend R. during Ayurveda Yoga Training, Berlin, 2018

The Yoga Sutras by Patanjali: An Attempt for Clarification of Used Terms

Nicholas Sutton's interpretations from the Oxford Hindu Studies Centre are used here for the original Sanskrit text. As it turned out, even close students of Shree Krishnamacharya, like his son, Desikachar, used interpretations that were often far from the original. I had happily been using the interpretations from Desikachar, as I liked his book in which he is an interesting conversation with a psychoanalyst. Only until Prof. Martin Mittwede pointed out: "Could you, please, read the original to me and then look at the interpretation?"

When I got aware that Desikachar has written long columns of text that had just nothing to do with the Sutra he was referring to!

Modern yoga would not exist without the dedicated work of Krishnamachrya. He has claimed that he discovered ancient yogic scriptures that introduced him to a unique yoga practice. His three, today's still most popular and influential, disciples were:

—B.K.S Iyengar, who established his style of precise Asana alignment and the use of props (specific tools that are helpful to achieve steadiness in a posture even without having the full physical capacity to do so) (Iyengar Yoga).

—Shri Patabhi Jois (the founder of Ashtanga Yoga practice, a standardised sequence-based practice), and

—Desikachar, Krishnamacharya's son, developed a gentle, individualised therapeutic style with psychological sensitivity called Vini—Yoga.

As we had discussed earlier in this book, Nicolas Sutton points out that the variations of the Sutras are vast as the absence of verbs allow in numerous translations or interpretations. So far, no one can claim the authorisation.

Patanjali and Samkhya: The Creation of the Universe, the Mahabhutas, Ahamkara and the Gunas

Why yoga and fundamentally Patanjali's yoga Sutras are used as a source for research into the darkness surrounding trauma patients?

Patanjali's Yoga and Ayurveda widely share the same source of theory about the creation of the universe, mind, matter and the Samkhya philosophy system however, focusing in opposite directions. Whereas in Shamkhya the unfolding of the Universe into the finest structures is described, yoga is the knowledge that all of this should be traced back to the original unity.

According to Samkhya Philosophy, there are three significant categories of mind and emotion:

- *Sattva,*
- *Raja,*
- *Tamas,*

as the 3 gunas or "qualities."(there are 20 more gunas as qualities of all kinds classified)

All set up in 3 other categories:

123

- *Manas,*
- *Citta,*
- *Buddhi,*

    as the faculties of the mind

Woven together by:

- *Ahamkara,*the ego—maker.

In the west, the *dosha* concept of ayurveda is famous as the central aspect and often the only known aspect of ayurveda. The *gunas* are not as widely used as an explanation for disease or insanity as the *doshas* are.

According to Samkhya, the *gunas* are widely translated as "mental *doshas*" which does not respect the differences in time in creation. The guna*s* appear earlier in creation and are not connected to matter (the *Tan Matras*) as the *doshas* are which consist of matter and subtle forces. Particularly, the action/non-action of *tamas* differ in yoga and ayurveda.

The following is my very own description and analysis of the three gunas in a psychiatric/psychological context of trauma. As there is not much research done so far, I was completely relying on the compliance of my patients and our dialectic approach on the journey of recovery. The following therefore has space for improvement and fresh evaluation.

Tamas

Traumatised patients and those with PTSD often adapt to their painful haunting past or even still present experiences by denial, dissociation, passiveness or inertia. Separation from the event or from their authentic self as the loss of connection describes the psychological term of dissociation. Dissociation is an experience where the patients lose connection with their bodily needs and feelings, their surrounding as environment, with their clarity of thoughts and judgment. Even a trance-like, sleepy state is described in one of the case studies.

Another way the patient tries to deal with the problem of depression and anxiety is through ignorance. Ignorance or denial is another attempt of the patients trying to deal with overwhelming feelings like anxiety, fear and arousal. This does not mean that those patients have an actual deficit or problem in logical understanding, learning or intelligence or that the patients are not sensitive, sensible or other.

But the ropes that tie them to the past resist any change despite knowing better (*Tamas*). They often feel as if they spend most of their time emotionally lost, being alone in darkness. A tendency to continue contributing to those (tamasic) feelings through the abuse of alcohol, through hoarding, drug abuse or internet distraction is always present and difficult to control—Avoidance of any change is just a slight hope for comfort. Change is a path into the uncomfortable unknown.

Some traumatised patients, like victims of domestic violence for example, often refuse to leave their daily horror as it often feels safer to know what to expect, to know the enemy than to move out and forward into an unpredictable new life. If nothing in life has ever been experienced as a safe place, it is hard to even imagine that a change could bring a new perspective and safety. If those patients manage to move out of their survival shell, they still have to face innumerable unwanted memories of the past that can pop up at any time and moment if triggered (arousal). The past infuses the present and the future on all levels, in the healthy being and more in those struggling with PTSD.

Rajas

Rajas can be another emotional response to distress. *Rajasic* responses occur more likely if the patient has enough stamina or their *prakriti* allows them to tap into the inborn power of *pitta*. *Rajas*, in the context of PTSD, is fighting. It can also be showing signs of psychopathic or narcissistic traits as both allow dominance over the other party with a lack of empathetic emotional involvement.

Fighting the memory and all connecting triggers becomes the dominating attitude of the survivor that affects personal relationships as much as daily life. In the context of trauma and PTSD, the dominant attitude towards life in general is exhausting. Driving a car to work can feel like being on a battlefield and one is not going to lose the competition! A hyper-alert state consumes all mental energies and leads to a tunnel vision that does not allow moderate or sensible answers.

Regular daily situations where patience is required might be experienced as a provocation and can end in an outbreak of uncontrolled anger or even violence. In this state, we often see ourselves as therapist being confronted with a victim and survivor who could have become a perpetrator himself.it is important at this point to be clear what our own limitations in therapy are. We have to understand what behaviour might be a trigger to us. What personal traits might cause us to end a therapeutic session?

It is helpful to monitor vital parameters like the Heartbeat rate and cortisol level to predict recovery. If the mind is agitated, scattered and aggressive, being in a state of hyper reaction to possible threats at all times, the muscles, particularly in the *pitta*-dominated region of the neck and shoulders, can be stiff and prone to injury. Patients suffering from constant pain in this area might be survivors of trauma and living in rajas. It is important to detect underlying painful memories to make the right treatment choice and avoid triggering aspects.

Treatment should include diligent learning how to control the mind. This is a chance to decide which memory will colour the future. Understanding the nature of the mind and the techniques to control, modify and alter the response to the distress, emotional onsets from the inside (memories) or outside (real experiences) can be acquired only by regular practice.

It is vital to prepare the patient that there is no immediate peak experience (which they search for) but a slight and constant decrease of unwanted emotions and an increase of moderate emotional responses to either memories or actual experiences. Slow happiness and meaning-making can instead be the responses to expect. Awareness, mindfulness and other meditative techniques can become essential tools to help the patient out of acute panic and arousal caused by unwanted memories. It is essentially for the therapist/patient relation to keep notes of any changes.

Sattva

There is a chance to live a life in tranquillity and happiness even for the traumatised patient. With good guidance and adequate individualised techniques to transform lifestyle and eating habits, selecting life's companions (partners, friends, a friendly surrounding) combined with diligent breathing practice and *asanas* from Patanjali's Eight Fold yoga Path to a safe space can be created.

However, sometimes drastic decisions and discipline might be needed to make a change. Nothing changes if nothing changes.

The Project "Massage, Meditation and Mindfulness" that I ran with Dr Anastasia Shchedrina and others, working with refugees from the Middle East (Syria, Yemen, Palestine, Iraq, Egypt) as well as with victims of domestic violence from Eastern Europe (Ukraine, Russia, Estonia):had focused on the message **the true home is only in yourself**.

The physical body can learn to experience a feeling of safety and home through meditation and touch. The safe space is the sattvic quality of the mind. However hard it is to regain the feeling of safety for traumatised patients, it is not impossible in the right setting. The often horrendous narratives of female refugees from Syria and Palestine included all cruelties a human being can experience by another human being yet still they reported benefit and relief during the exercises on meditation, massage and mindfulness and even long-lasting effects after the project.

A feeling of home and safe space restoration will eventually increase resilience, lead to recovery and might slowly even achieve healing. The victim—self might eventually disappear and the free person, the original self, can emerge. This is what we call "Healing from Trauma."

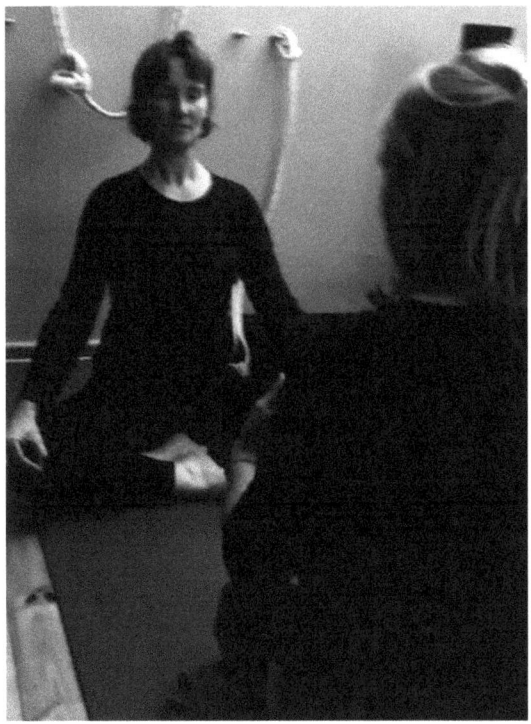

Photo: the author. Student R. performing the above pose under direct instructions of her student friend M. during Ayurveda Yoga Training, Berlin, 2018

Table: Behavioural and Psychological Manifestation of *Tri Guna*

The table is an attempt to display a rough overview of the psychological factors described as the *gunas (http://Charakasamhitaonline.com/mediawiki title Unmada Nidana, seen on 13.05.2020).*

Sattva	Rajas	Tamas
Enlightening	Propulsive and dynamic	Inhibitive
Efforts for more knowledge	Overexpression of pain and pleasure	Ignorant
Theism (appreciates the existence of Almighty	Active	Excessive fatigue of sense organs
Straight forward dealing	Industrious	Atheism
Polite	Egoistic	Inactive
Gratitude	Reacting	Poor
Of good memory, intellect	Angry	More sleep
Prompt to learn	Pretender	Worrying
Serious	Jealous	Commits mistakes
Welfare wisher	Brave	Unhygienic
	Greedy	.
	Cruel	
	Tense	

The Yoga Sutras as a guide on the road of healing. Thoughts, observations and trials from my therapeutic work.

I.1 *Atha yoganushasanam*
Here or now begins the instruction to yoga.

There is a discussion about the Atha: as it can be translated as here or now. There is nothing before. Everything ends and something new starts.

I.2 *Yogash cittavrittinirohah*

Nicolas Sutton translates this: yoga is the restriction of the movements of the mind. Sutton introduces Citta as a thinking faculty. He explains that the term mind, widely used as translation, is "p*robably as close as we can get in English.*" Interesting enough, in my mother tongue German there is no equivalent for the word *mind* existing.

The word vritti is translated as movement, it is an activity. If we connect the words citta and vritti, as in cittavritti, we describe the movement of the thoughts, the wavering, the loops, the content. There is content of what we want to think but we all know, content of what we truly do not want to think. The famous example: do not think of polar bears leads to an endless loop of polar bears appearing on the inner screen. With this example, we realise the content of the thoughts is not in our hands. However, the restriction of the process is.

This clear, direct and straightforward paragraph explains the functions of the mind and what can be achieved by practicing yoga. Practicing the real yoga is yoga self-explaining. Yoga is not a subject but merely an experience that is carried out through reflected actions and the benefits and virtues of mind (citta) control.

It is a common assumption in psychiatry that in the case of psychological trauma, the memory of the incident is immediately neglected and suppressed— or the opposite could be true, too: the memory gets obsessively repeated, depending on the school of psychiatry.

According to Patanjali's explanation, the traumatic injury might not be the problem but the repeated memory of the actions, surroundings, smells, fear, helpers or no help after the incident. However, through practice, the memory can eventually redirect into less disturbing figures. The patients can actively learn to move on by focusing on the direction they are going from now on instead of looking back.

There is no possible recovery from trauma and PTSD for a scattered mind, however the scattered mind can be healed. The repetitive experience of arousals as an emotional response to similar distress (sound, smell, location, date, etc.) can overwhelm the patient at any time or place. It can be caused by other peoples' narratives and memories of the same or another traumatising event during group sessions, even if there is no real-time can cause one to feel the same way.

Generations of Holocaust survivors carry our painful burden within collective memory and so do Palestinian families who would do anything to finally receive a safe passport and try to break the chain of pain and fear The scars of hundreds of years of war have formed the brain of survivors of endless conflicts, war and other threats to life like famine, drought and its stressor centres in a particular way of higher distress response.

Traumatic events are mostly not inert singularities and trajectories encourage a longer post-trauma time perspective than often expected. Immediate responses to stress are not the only indicators of adjustment to constant stress exposure; more important is the eventual and ultimate resolution of the stressful event through mind control.

The traumatised person's mind has learned from the traumatising experience and filters memory during and after the traumatic event, tinting everything that gets close to the initial stress—if the *citta* does not learn to eradicate the fluctuations of the mind. The mind draws conclusions and would change behaviour by either giving up hope and not seeing a future that makes it worth living or learns to find peace and happiness through introducing the victim to positive experiences.

Unfortunately, learning from the traumatising event can be a repetition of stored memory content (from the *manas* and *citta)*. Even when a patient reports that she cannot remember anything from their shocking experience, they still retain the emotions of distress at the time and immediately after the event. However, many of the actual event memories might turn out to be false or falsified memories.

Famous stories of false memories of threats highlight the situation that memory is more complex than thought. The filter of personal experience amplifies each memory. Memory is only created in crude mode and is easy to manipulate, model or modify. In trauma/PTSD, it is like the repetition of the meaningless sound of a broken record. However, the memory is not fading. It does disappear over time. It can sleep. As neuroscience discovered, each time the stored memory is requested through a triggering aspect, its contents get fully refreshed.

As Aristotle said: *the memory is like a stamp on running water.*

A patient (survivor of the Berlin Christmas Market attack) reported that she cannot remember the actual impact of the truck or the moment of the breaking down of stalls where she was standing and what precisely she saw or heard at the very moment. Instead, she remembers finding herself in a different location, wondering how she possibly ended up there. There was clearly a gap in her narrative.

However, she clearly remembers fear, smells and images of dying and injured victims. The reaction got stored. The disgust, nausea, fear and being exposed to an unsafe environment can turn on hell in the mind without the slightest warning. The memory of the direct impact, though, is unclear. Yet any memory is open to manipulation.

In the chapter on The Memory Illusion: Where were You When 9/11 Happened? Julia Shaw presents several different theories on the mind and memory. Striking is her story about an incident during the Vietnam war. A person was accused of lying several years after he had made his story of survival public. It had turned out that he was actually on the scene much later in a safe place, but hearsay and witnessing some parts of the actual incident created a false memory.

However, his symptoms and the content of the memory were true in the sense that they were absolutely true to him. Important notice here: the above information should never put a victim's memory into discredit as such but also not take all the information as a proof of the traumatic impact.

These days we see a growing number of patients seeking help with Ayahuasca or other psychedelic drugs, taking the upcoming pictures as a content of a hidden memory and as a proof. But, as we saw earlier, there is no proof of an emotional experience. Hallucinogenic drugs will not reveal any other truth than the memory that is stored, but we now know that the stored memory is most likely a fluent pattern of several faculties of the mind, open to change and retelling, influence and loss.

However, the symptoms and reactions of the victim are the truth for us as therapists. Here, atha, here and now we start. Why did we look into this? Because we also see now clearly that any content of the memory and the reaction towards it can be changed.

Yet the most exciting information from the above is: memory traces can be changed.

The standard examination after a traumatic event through police or health workers often influences the memory of the victims or witnesses. It even affects the memory for later on. The way an interrogator asks a question can influence the focus of the memory and answer and, therefore, the stored memory. After a synagogue attack by a truck in Tunisia, police asked the survivors a simple question: did the truck have the lights on? Was the truck blue?

By asking these particular questions, they created a memory. Commonly, it is not remembered if cars have their lights on. The question suggests that the lights were on and about 80 per cent of the survivors and witnesses then reported: yes, the lights were on! And the truck was blue as this information was already included in the question and therefore memorised. It is impossible, as we all know the famous example, not to think of pink polar bears!

Therefore, therapists, who ask questions about the nature of the trauma and specific memories have to strictly avoid involuntary manipulating. In yoga, we discover a completely different solution to the dilemma: no questions at all.

Yoga with the aim of controlling the movement of *Citta* is a clear way to experience the *now* instead of finding traces in the past. The actual presence of the moment shared directs attention towards it. Nevertheless, it is not a strategy to simply ignore the past. To live with the past means to integrate the experiences and direct the mind into the present.

According to the translation of the Yoga—Sutras of Patanjali by Swami Veda Bharati, Vyasa's commentary says that yoga is the control of the modifications of the mind-field. And he continues explaining that the 3 disposition of the mind field as the following: illumination as *pra-khya* from *sattva*, endeavour as in *pra-vrtti* from *rajas* and stasis as in *sthiti* from *tamas.*

Different to general western textbooks which declare *tamas* a function with a lack of positive qualities, all Indian sources that are based on the classics are clearly seeing the necessities of a tamasic quality, represented here in the term *stithi,* which is not only stasis but stability.

In western texts, we find mostly words like inability to learn, stubborn, lazy which does not reflect the virtue of stability and consistency. We do see here a problem of transferring knowledge, if authors tend to interpret according to their own cultural context. If we want to use the knowledge of yoga for healing complex PTSD, we have to address the absence of good tamasic qualities in our society as a problem. Only in stages of trauma that are characterised by a lack of Vata and Pitta, sattva and rajas, focusing on tamas as *stithi* would be a fundamental mistake. It is the drop of oil that makes the wheel run smoothly, but too much oil solidifies and blocks.

I.11 *Anubhuta-vishaya-sampramoshah smritih*

Experiences can be retained in the memory.

Memory is stored in *manas*. It is said *manas* is like a film projector that projects the memories on the screen of *citta* where it can be seen. The memory bank *citta* then is clouding the moment by interpreting it from the past. Therefore, it is characterised by selective cognition and leads to false assumptions.

In Trauma, a triggering aspect of memory (like the smell of burnt sugar-coated almonds from the Christmas Market) can become a reliving momentum of the event: arousal, which describes the onset of a cascade of fear, anxiety, an increase of heartbeat rate, panic attack, etc. By achieving control of our memory's content, the patient will realise the actual state they are in, the present and the accurate surrounding instead of an interpretation of the moment by the mind, repeating a situation from the past.

I.30 vyaadhi-*styaana-sanshaya-pramaadaalasyaavirati-bhranti-darashanaalabdha-bhuumikatvanavasthitatvaani citta-vikshepaas te 'ntarayah*
The interpretation is the following: disease, doubt, denial, indulgence, misapprehension, laziness, lack of consistency indolence and flakiness that are the obstacles that keep the mind from steadiness.

As in western yoga practice primarily *asanas* and *pranayama* are performed and physical fitness is often the focus, traditional yoga rooted in yoga philosophy can establish faith and mental clarity by setting achievable goals for everyone, not depending on physical fitness but on inner motivation and the will to change and diligence.

The therapist, however, should be cautious not to set the goals too high which can often be seen in toxic positivity goals as frustration and negative thinking will doubtlessly be the result. Those goals should not be set too low as well as too quick achievement without overcoming difficulties will not increase resilience. If the standard is low, a feeling of failure, thought of as incompetent, inferior or lazy, can destroy the patient/therapist relationship.

The patient whose *rajas* dominates will not feel acknowledged but devaluated, as the therapist assumes that the patient cannot do something of greater value. The self-doubt of the patient often arises from low self-esteem. The covert narcissist is a good example of a difficult patient/therapist relationship in rajas.

The Five Kleshas

The five *Kleshas* are often translated as significant obstacles on the path of self-realisation. They explain the influence of false identification and fear as root problems of every personality.

1. *Avidya*: Ignorance

The first Klesha shows disconnection from the truth and a lack of self-awareness.

Mistaking pain for pleasure is an example that most people can relate to. Patients with PTSD often find themselves in unhappy and abusive relationships, which they justify by focusing on what they think they gain from it. Another example is the use of alcohol and recreational drugs, which result in assumptions of false truth and pleasure.

One patient had commented: "Addiction is the false door to connection." The pleasure that had been looked for deceases quickly and leaves the patient in a mentally and physically weaker position than before. *Avidya* conditions the mind through repetitive behaviour to escape the unwanted experiences and memories physically without allowing the mind to educate itself and recover by focusing on the positive outcome on the mental level.

2. *Asmita*: Ego

Ego is not a bad quality at all, it is often mistaken as an almost evil force in some western yoga schools—Ego defines, separates. It separates the I from the You. Many western yoga students often mistake ego as a flaw one has to overcome. Ego is a very efficient protective shield as it defines borders—when it is healthy, *ahamkara,* creates the *I*.

It is important to see a difference in the world between the " I " and the others. As Swami Satchitananda from Bihar School of Yoga commented that" One first has to understand the differences before one can see the union." (Bihar School of Yoga). The ego of a traumatised person often shattered. If a person gets traumatised at a time of her life before the *ahamkara* fully unfolds, the false self might take its place. Such a person is prone to develop psychological symptoms or even schizophrenia. As one patient said: "Me and my daughter are ONE."

This is not a psychologically healthy state of ego. Mother and daughter are separate people and personalities with their own faith. Her daughter would probably have disagreed. The patient herself had significant issues with her mother. Her mother had abandoned her as a child while out partying and left her with strangers. Therefore, the Ego should be used as a tool for inquiring the world and dropped when it comes to self-inquiry.

3. *Raga*: Attachment

Raga is defined as desire or possessiveness. The desire to possess includes relations, objects, friends and goals. Clinging to things of desire results in pain, grief and anger. If *rajas* is involved, the person cannot let go of desire or expectations as it might feel like losing control. The mind considers the objects of desire as permanent and is clouded to see the impermanence. Desire become affliction and addiction and causes suffering.

After a short-term pleasure, one has to face the long-term consequences. Attachment is a life force, too. Attachment creates family bonds and drives societies. Attachment is of different values to each individual, but the result is always suffering. A common adaption of survivors with Compulsive Behaviour Disorder displays the absurdness of clinging and controlling objects to experience security. However, all objects are just temporary.

4. *Dvesha*: Aversion

Aversion is the other face of desire. All desired objects or relations lose their fascination over time. After some time, they all taste stale. The always wondering *citta*—mind moves from one pole to the other, from attachment to aversion and aversion to attachment.

Not only pleasurable and desired thoughts and situations are repetitively reoccurring in the memory and but also memories that create aversion. The mind has no power of discrimination and *citta* does not decide about the moral or quality of the thought. Even the most unpleasant thought triggered by attachment, as in the case of trauma: the memory of the unwanted situation comes back because there is mental detachment.

At the same time, aversion happens: the patient tries to reject the thought. All the energy that goes into the aversion becomes an attachment. Therefore, the repetition of favourable moments is important until the memory as *citta* where the *Vrittis* reach a peaceful equilibrium. It is impossible to study *raga* without *Dvesha* and vice versa.

5. ***Abhinivesha***:

Clinging to life. It is often translated as: the fear of death.

A lot of impulsive decisions are made because of the fear of death. Jumping to assumptions that life is short and one should indulge as much, no regrets, stop the patient from truly living life to its fullest.

Quotes like *You live only once.* are misguiding the traumatised and confused person into a harmful lifestyle. A life filled with excuses and self-deception. It often starts with excuses covered up in sayings like: *I deserve this. Everything was so difficult today. I now deserve it.* This self-excusing mindset of unaware, ignorant behaviour is seen in all *doshas* with different main topics. Examples:

- In the case of *Kapha*: "I can eat this now. I deserve it. I don't have to follow these rules. I need comfort. I deserve it now."
- In the case of *Vata*: "I don't need rest. I can go out and stay up late. I deserve the distraction. I can start this, I can spend the money. I deserve this."
- In the case of *Pitta*: "I can take these drugs/money, have sex with whom I want. I am the centre of the world. I deserve this to let off some steam."

It is important to explain and reveal the patterns of self-damaging behaviour to the patient in a subtle and friendly way. Telling a patient off for particular coping behaviour might cause the opposite: the patient might feel mothered or patronising in a negative sense—the best learning effect is the one that creates positive feelings, gratitude and self-esteem.

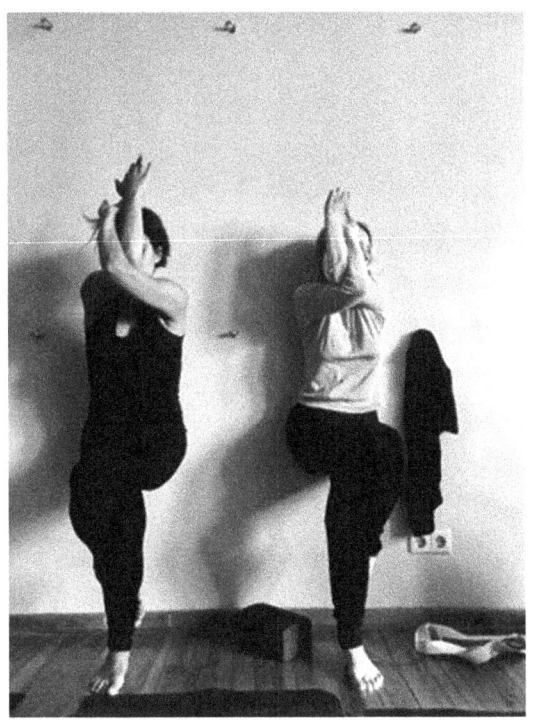

Photo: the author. Two students are performing, supported Garudasana against the wall. By doing so, they experience stability and reach a focused state more easily. First, they study the *asana* standing freely in the room. Inevitably, they move and shake. Then, the practice against the wall allows precise alignment correction. After integrating the new experience, they move into an unsupported stand again, incorporating the experienced stability and staying focused. Students M. and N. during Ayurveda Yoga Teacher Training at Society of Friends, Berlin, 2018

The Yoga Sutras as a Guideline for Self-Inquiry

The complex and structured system of understanding the mind and its functions through studying *Samkhya* philosophy offers a deep insight into the interwoven functions of the sensory organs, consciousness and memory. The 3 *gunas* direct the healing approach. Each *guna* that is dominant in a patient permanently will result in different treatment approaches. Without the quality of *Rajas, Sattva* cannot become an authentic quality. *Rajas* and *sattva* together are necessary to overcome *tamas*. In other words:

If trauma has become the crucial part of negative assumptions of the patients' lives, they have lost the *guna* of *Sattva*, of inner peace. From there, pain and suffering are arising, opening two roads: the *guna* of *Rajas* can create such pain that the patient longs for peace and is ready to overcome life's obstacles to heal. *Tamas,* however, the quality of inertia is like a pain killer. It does not allow the patient to feel, instead being in hibernation and dissociation. There will be no development, only denial.

It is important to understand that the *gunas* are not "either/or" components of being. They are the very qualities of everything, yet different objects differ in their qualities and the human mind and consciousness. In case of trauma, a severe change took place and had thrown the *gunas* out of their equilibrium. Through the initiation to *pranayama (breath control)* during yoga therapeutic settings, the patient experiences *sattva* again.

Yoga provides a detailed executive plan about knowledge of the *Citta, Buddhi, Ahamkara* and the *gunas* and how to achieve insight and change. Yoga is a way to inquire how to overcome false assumptions and live a life by revealing the inner truth.

Through refined techniques of *pranayama* (directing breath) and *Asanas* (postures) as well as techniques of *Pratyahara* (withdrawal of the senses) and *Dhyana* (Meditation), combined with ayurveda which adds the greatness of touch, feeling and taste can help the patient to reunite the "body-mind" continuum.

This book was written during the countries' Corona (Covid-19) lockdown. The curfew was an extremely difficult time particularly for victims of domestic violence, refugees and many other traumatised patients. However, the frequent daily online contact with me as a therapist and the practice that happened online in one-to-one sessions and even group sessions of *pranayama* or *asana* classes have shown tremendous helpful support through *Dinacharya*.

The daily regimen of patients had successfully supported them in creating meaning-making and reduced the significant onset of major depressive disorders in many ways. The progress in their overall (positive perspective) feeling towards life that they can achieve through daily *pranayama* is satisfying. The alterations of the stress response through Yoga *Asana* and *pranayama* as well as Meditation time spent in a safe space helped to build a stable foundation practice for the time after.

Therapy and the Way Out: Different Models to Transform Experiences of Trauma Into Individual Narratives of Hope and Recovery

Western Psychiatric and Psychologic Therapy Models for Trauma and PTSD

According to the different concepts on understanding trauma in general (psychiatric, neurobiological, psychological, genetic, neurological and others) very few therapy strategies meet the individuality of patient's response to trauma like PTSD and other psychiatric or psychological problems. The traumatic event itself is the medical classification itself to find a suitable trauma informed therapist who then decides about the treatment according to their education, not necessarily to the type of person who experienced the trauma, their cultural, gender, socio-political or other background.

However, not many of the traumatised patients I saw in my clinic in the last 40 years have ever been diagnosed with trauma before. This is often due to the inability of their GPs to diagnose trauma as the underlying condition of their various health issues or it's due to the patient's inability to ask for help or the patient does not see a problem in their life as their compensative and adaptive behaviour might have built a tight fence around any emotional insight into the past events.

Various adaptive patterns to trauma like poly-toxic drug/alcohol/pain medication abuse, auto—or general aggressive behaviour, addiction and depression, eating disorders, gambling, porn binging or other are often not considered part of the trauma treatment. Due to their complexity, they might require extra specialists or clinical care.

However, a few of the new treatment methods listed below are promising.

Various new trauma informed therapies were developed in the last decades to deal with repeated stress events and PTSD. Some of them are listed here. In addition to the classical therapies, such as Freud's psychoanalysis and psychotherapy of classical schools (Jung, Adler), the following modern approaches are now widely used and some of them are already part of Germany's social insurance coverage:

- 1. Eye Movement Desensitisation and Reprocessing (EMDR)
- 2. Short term Therapy (IS-TDP)
- 3. Brain spotting

- 4. Somatic Experience (SE)
- 6. Neurolateral Imaginative Trauma Therapy (NLITT)
- 7. Interapy
- 8. Virtual Reality Therapy
- 9. Emotional Freedom Technique (EFT)
- 10. Narrative Psychotherapy
- 11. Trauma-sensitive Yoga Therapy

Definitions and Methods of some of the Recent Developed Therapies:

1. EMDR

Therapy method developed by Francine Shapiro in Palo Alto, California. Eye movement and desensitisation and reprocessing are the key terms. The central point is an induced rapid eye movement during the remembrance of traumatic contents. The theory states that this results in bilateral brain stimulation and leads to fading memory of the traumatic injury itself. Bilateral stimulation of the brain could be achieved by finger tapping on the thighs, following a moving finger with the eyes or other auditory or tactile stimulants.

2. ISTDP

Intensive Psychodynamic Short-Term Therapy. Davanloo developed this therapy in two versions:
as short-term therapy or in an analytical version (Major Mobilisation of the Unconscious and Psychoanalytical Investigation).
An analysis of filmed sessions with the patients allowed the patients to open up to early emotions and overcome fear and resistance. The direct physical reliving of archaic emotions is considered key to dissociated traumatic childhood trauma. Change of character, consequent change of relationship patterns and constant symptom healing are the goal.

3. Brainspotting

Brainspotting, developed in 2003, took the experience from Somatic Experience and EMDR Opposite to EMDR, Grand, the founder of Brain spotting, believes that a fixed eye movement or a specific eye fixation would help processing traumatic memories. The idea is similar to EMDR Conscious remembrance offers an option to reconsider and finally forget the contents of traumatic memory.

While doing so, the patient must be aware and name or show the body parts in which they feel the most activity during reinforced memory. The therapist moves freely with his hand in the patient's visual field until the patient loses track of the movement, which is considered a brain spot. The patient is then encouraged of awareness on their effects, memory, cognition and bodily sensations to keep focused. The distress level from 1 to 10 allows the therapist to consider the treatment as successful. So far, research shows lower effectivity than EMDR.

4. Somatic experience is a body-oriented approach to healing trauma and other stress disorders. Created by Dr Peter Levine and considered a multidisciplinary study of stress physiology, psychology, ethology, biology, neuroscience, indigenous healing practices and medical biophysics.

All newer therapies (compared to psychanalysis, psychotherapy based on speaking) start with the assumption that trauma shows signs of cognitive impairment, therefore therapies that consider healing through re-cognition are less effective than those that are experience based. Experiences of traumatic triggering contexts can be harmful in my eyes. The focus of the broken narrative oppose to starting fresh is based on the cultural understanding of time as a linear process differing from that most Oriental cultures see time as a circle.

"Somatic Experience": The Empirical Treatment Approach by Bessel Van der Kolk, Gabor Mate and Peter Levine

Two leading names in treating PTSD are Bessel Van der Kolk and, more popular to the public, Peter Levine. Necessary for this research study is their current therapy approach through what they call "somatic experience". Levine is convinced that the traumatic experience shocks the brain, freezes the body and stuns the mind.

In my understanding, we take those sentences in and tend to agree quickly, without really clarifying the terms, particularly the term mind. In this description, the whole of the 3 faculties of a person are altered. He then continues by mentioning the impact on the memory of the body, brain and mind, from there to psyche and soul. He states that the healer loses her or his way in the labyrinth of cause and effect. We are here confronted again with total of a shattered being, where there is nothing left and that healers show to be incompetent by the vast range of destruction.

This is much in contrast to our experiences, where we actually focus on the remaining structures: what is enduring? What are the distinct qualities of strength in that particular person? Where is the joy, where the joyful memories?

Somatic experience has become a landmark among the currently available therapy solutions for trauma patients. The US-American homepage for PTBS victims, the US Department of Veterans Affairs, suggests that soldiers first try psychological therapies and only then, if still needed, start with pharmacotherapy *(2017 VA/DoD Clinical Practice Guideline for PTBS)*.

This is a significant recent breakthrough in the treatment of PTSD. The patients are advised first to seek non-drug help instead of the expected standard of sedating the patients so that they do not feel the pain. The alarmingly fast-growing numbers in the US of opiate-addicted patients might have contributed to the change of concepts.

In addition to "somatic experience," many other so called "holistic" concepts have been applied to trauma therapy. A growing number of treatments under the name "Trauma Therapy" are available in alternative medicine centres and bits of ayurveda or Chinese Medicine concepts are taken out of their historical and truly holistic context to develop a "new treatment approach." "Trauma" seems to be merely the wheel reinvented.

It represents the recent rediscovery of psychological distress that was discovered 80 years ago—when back then there was no understanding of the short and long-term changes that could take place in a patient.

Thanks to the dedicated studies of Levine and Van der Kolk, an understanding of psycho-physiological responses to traumatic events is happening now. However, a big drawback of Van der Kolk's and Levine's work in my eyes is that their research and their trauma therapy approach was focused mainly on traumatised soldiers.

Overly relying on data from studies on soldiers is problematic for trauma studies because the knowledge gained from studying soldiers' experiences has been uncritically transferred on all other trauma sufferers without considering potentially important differences. While soldiers experience several different stress factors and different aftercare to victims of domestic violence, witnesses of terror attacks, raped members of the LGTBQ+ community, refugees and others, soldiers knowingly enter a potentially traumatising environment.

Surrounded by brothers-in-arms who are most likely to experience similar distress. They are somewhat prepared for the traumas of war and trained to defend themselves. Unlike soldiers, most refugees, genocide, abused children, victims of domestic violence or other trauma survivors are seldom surrounded by people who will experience similar distress during their exposure, having had no training for self—defence or even a chance to escape.

They mostly did not have the opportunity to be repatriated, cared for or brought to a safe space on time. They are less likely to receive a public honour for their pain. Living in a country that had accepted thousands of refugees from Syria but had no plan to care for them, not even a safe place for women and children during their long times in camps.

In my eyes, more studies are urgently needed to understand the more diverse pictures of trauma experience of the individual and of the after math. Victims from the overly represented groups of survivors of trauma like POC (people of colour), LGTBQ+ (lesbian, gay, trans, bi, queer and other) immigrants, refugees, disabled, children display distinct support requirements.

Based on my clinical study on complementary healing with ayurveda and yoga I see that these provide unexpected and precise answers to the western science-dominated medical world when it comes to the explanation what happened and how can we continue to deal with the traumatic experience, the changes and adaptions on an individualised way—

However, the diagnosis of Trauma in the west is a generalisation which is represented as a medical diagnosis under the catalogue of diagnostic categories for insurance purposes. It does not necessarily lead to an individualised treatment plan that considers individual factors, like childhood sexual assault, terror attacks, victims of war, etc. Unfortunately, no plans to correct personal lifestyle of the victim and offer holistic experiences like keeping a proper daily routine, healthy individual nutrition, adapted exercise and a perspective in life through meaning-making.

By cutting bits out of traditional healing systems like Ayurveda, Oriental Medicine, Yoga, there is an actual loss of connection towards a complex system of a priori beliefs, meaning and procedures for the individual and the society, family and network in which the trauma occurred.

Ayurveda's way of faith: Treatments for Cittodvega and Unmada
A critical attempt of adaption to the use of the western terms of Trauma and PTSD

Ayurveda has an uncountable variety of treatment options according to the uncountable variety of conditions of the patient, the family, the social network around the patient, the individual experience and the reaction to incidents, only to name a few important factors.

So correctly spoken, the number of ayurveda treatment plans are the exact number of patients—as each patient is treated with an individualised treatment plan.

However, there are few specific treatments described. Besides the diagnosis of the current complaints, the cause of the disease matters as much as the adaption to the cause. A differentiation is made, for example, if the disease is *Adhaytmika*, means karmic, that affects the mind and the consciousness and can be named. This is often only translated into congenital defects. But *Adhidaivivka* includes seasonal problems in the diagnosis, like a monsoon, wind or even *physical and psychological derangement caused by supernatural or natural events and disasters* (Lingham,2015), which would fit into a modern description of a traumatic experience.

In the context of this book, however, there will be only a brief overview of optional treatment methods and only Shirodhara is extensively explained.

Dravya Guna: The Indian Pharmacopeia of Herbs and Substances

Indian Pharmacopeia is not easily accessible. Written down as an encyclopaedia of herbs in hundreds of different languages it is even for the Indian scientist or researcher difficult to name them all, classify them and see the differences in approach towards health.

Again, the variety of climate, epochs, philosophical background, experiences and much more matter even in the use and preparation of a single plant—together with multiple other unknown factors like formulas that have been developed in some private practices and handed over to the next generation, written in languages only a few people would still speak. However, there are many specific herbs that the northern path of ayurveda and the southern path agree to.

Quite commonly, herbal formulas are prescribed. Brahmi (Bacopa monniera) and Ashvagandha (Withania somnifera) are the most used herbs for minor irritations. Both provide an increased ability to focus.

A major herb for the agitated mind is Jatamansi (Nardostachys jatamansi) which is not available anymore as the demand for it and the poorer harvest due to climate change contributed that the herb is almost extinct in the wild—It is now under international conservation. (Bose, Tripathy 2018)

The most widely used for PTSD, stress, Unmada, Cittodvega is Brahmi (bacopa monniera) as well as Mandukaparni which is also named Brahmi or Gotu Kola. In combination with milk or ghee, their uses are for madness/insanity, skin diseases, epilepsy/seizures, hoarseness of the throat, speech purification, for a good memory, as well as given for signs of possession/psychological damage. One to two teaspoons of churna (finely ground powder)should be taken 2-3 times a day, cooked in milk (Lingham,2015)(Glimpse of Mental Disorders and Treatment of Ayurveda).

An exceptional range of medical formulas for treating *Cittodvega/nmada* are Rasaushadhis. They are a very particular group of medical preparations, using heavy metal like mercury, lead or gold in combination with plants like Shankhapushbi (Evolvulus alsinoides), Jatamansi (Nardostachys jatamansi), Tagara (Valeriana indica), raisins like Shilajeet (Bitumen), Shallaki (Boswella serrata) and often ghee.

These prescriptions are banned from import to Europe. Despite the extensive procedures of detoxifying the heavy metals through specific processes, like cooking in milk, slow cooking them for weeks or months in clay pots in the soil and many more they often still contain a certain amount of toxic lead, arsenic or mercury (studies Sunday Naturals, 2016, Fresenius institute, private investigation).

However, investigating the used plants from the ancient days till nowadays formulas is challenging. Possible treatments in Europe differ significantly from those in India as the rules, bans and regulations on importing plants to Europe and use them as so-called novel food, medicine or spices makes it impossible to redesign the traditional formulas.

As in Europe and other countries, most of the suggested readymade remedies are not available and or, if, in poor quality. The focus on Dravya Guna (plant action, pharmacopeia) for the west should be based on the practicability of ayurvedic treatments in Europe and other countries. Some therapists aim to replace traditionally used Indian herbs with European medical plants. However, there is not much experience and clearly not an experience of 2500 years behind it.

Ayurveda Treatments Using Tailam, (medicated oil preparations)

Ayurveda uses medicated oils for a wide variety of indications. Medicated oils are oil preparations that often contain dozens of different plants, minerals, pastes, decoctions, infusions and often animal products like milk, ghee or urine.

Abhyanga, famous in the west as THE Ayurveda oil massage, is a way to slowly apply medicine in the form of oil the body. It is not a form of massage as Swedish or deep tissue massage, in fact Abhyanga avoids all pressure on the tissues.

An Abhyanga is a procedure of often 1-3 hours during which warm oil (thailam) enhanced with certain medical properties is applied to the body in defined strokes, often from 2 therapists simultaneously. Man massage man, women, massage women.

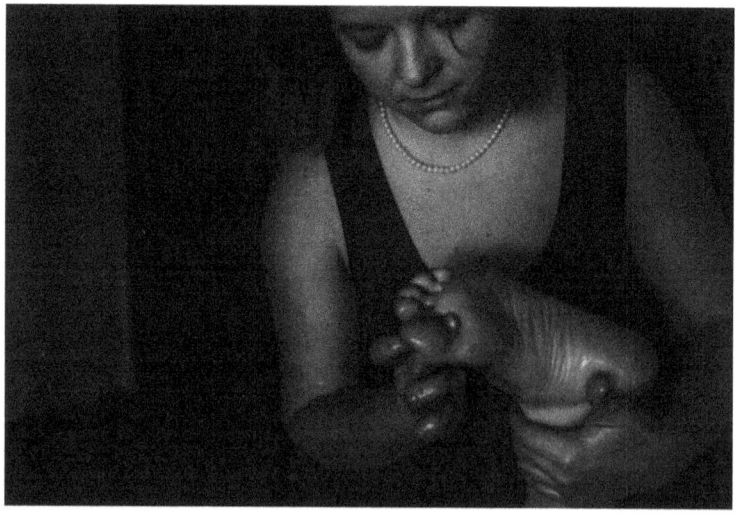

Photo: Dr Anastasia Shchedrina performing *pad abhyanga* (foot massage) on a patient, photo credit Natalia Smirnova, 2019

Another way to apply medicated oil is an intensified treatment called Shirodhara where oil is applied directly on the forehead, through constant pouring.

Shirodhara: The Olation of the Forehead

Shirodhara is another medical ayurveda procedures to calm the mind (*Citta*), pacify *Vata* and *Pitta*, clear the openings of the head (Shalakhyatantra) and eyes and reduce *Cittodvega* and *Unmada*—t is meant to reduce symptoms like sleeplessness, anxiety, panic attacks, high or very low blood pressure, self-harming behaviour.

It became one of the most popular procedures that are performed in the west, almost a symbol for ayurveda, printed on posters of advertisement. However, mostly unfortunately and even dangerously, considered a wellness treatment without any prescription or medical supervision. As a result, we saw traumatic arousals during the Shirodhara application, dissociation and even an increase of anxiety and panic that could even last for months.

According to the science of the *doshas,* it increases Kaphaja. Shirodhara can lead to a *sattvic mind* state, which translates as a method to decrease sympathetic responses and allow parasympathetic governed deep relaxation, proper sleep, decreased BP and pulse rate, harmonising mental attitude and a decrease of the fight and flight response.

Confirming all the above the studies at Society of Friends, Berlin, Shirodhara applications had reduced stress symptoms like anxiety, depression, high blood pressure, sleeplessness, aggression and panic attacks but we had to carefully chose the patients, monitor them before, during and after the application.it was important to build trust and a connection with the therapist first, before the patients were able to safely hand themselves over into the trancelike, dreamlike state.

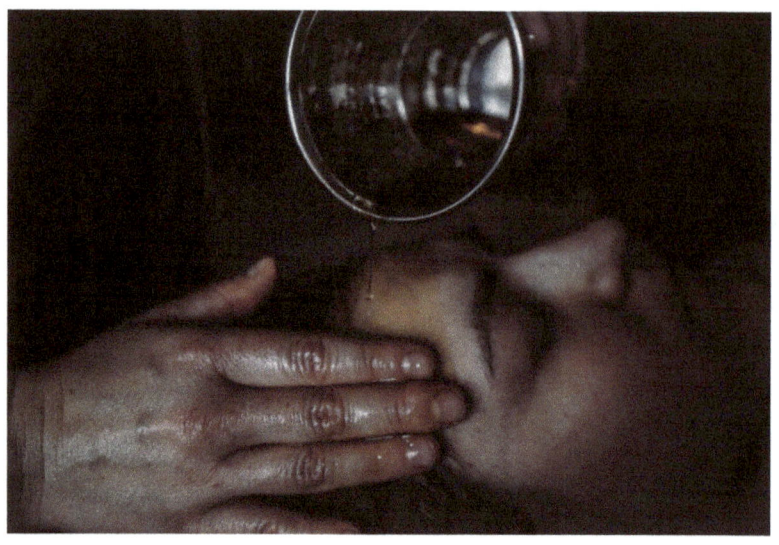

General Information of the Procedure of Shirodhara

Shirodhara is a Sanskrit word consisting of *Shiro*, the head and *Dhara*, the flow.

For the procedure, the patient is preferably placed on a wooden table.

In India, the different types of wood for each *dosha* are essential for a successful treatment. However, in western countries, the patients generally prefer a soft and slightly warmed up surface to lie on. One must consider that the effect might change due to the electrical field created by standard heated blankets.

The patient should be covered with a cotton veil or a thin blanket to keep the body warm, as relaxation might cool it down quickly. A particular head rest with a ditch to allow the oil to flow into a bowl is generally added to the massage table. Under the spout of the headrest are a set of clean bowls placed to silently receive the used oil.

In a distance of approximately 20-30 cm, a copper or stainless steel, clay or brass pot is hanging right above the centre of the patient's forehead. The vessel, often made of clay, copper, brass or stainless steel, can be used. Traditionally one up to three cotton threads are hanging out of the vessel's centre, but there is also a range of *Yantras* or spouts, available to alter the width and speed of the flow.

Depending on the *dosha* aggravation, the threads measure in numbers and length. For easier use and to provide a constant flow of either medicated oil or *Takra*, a buttermilk liquid, vessels with spouts that screw easily regulate the flow at any time and according to the patient's needs. The *Yantras* are easy to interrupt the flow of oils if the patient feels discomfort.

The medicated oil or Takra (buttermilk) is heated just above blood temperature. Some vessels even provide an adjustable thermostat to keep a steady temperature.

Commonly pre-cooked, so-called "matured" sesame oil is used for the Shirodhara. In addition, according to *dosha* imbalances, individually selected herbs can be cooked in oil, filtered and used.

Ashvagandhadi thailam or *Balathailam* are used to reduce anxiety and sleeplessness from aggravated *Vata Dosha*, *Bhringraja*thailam or *keram* is used to increase hair growth, *Brahmi, Mandukaparni or Shankhapushpi* are often used to calm an aggravated *Pitta Dosha*. Instead of using oil for high *Pitta* with aggression and high blood pressure symptoms, *takra* (buttermilk) mixed with herbs is preferably used.

Kseerabala Thailam (oil) is a special oil formula for increased *Vata—Pitta Dosha*. However, the prices of these medicated oils are high in India and elsewhere, which leads to the unfortunate situation that most therapists use plain sesame oil.

The patient's eyes are covered with cotton eye pads, soaked in rosewater. The ears partially blocked from all surrounding sounds with oil-soaked cotton buds. The forehead is protected at the eyebrow region with a thin cotton string to prevent oil from dripping into the eye sockets.

The Shirodhara starts after a short gentle. It also reduces symptoms like sleeplessness, anxiety, panic attacks, high or very low blood pressure, self-harming behaviour. *Abhyanga* of the shoulders, neck and face.

According to the patient's clinical symptoms and the number of applications, the time set for each treatment is between seven minutes up to two hours. The application time in India is usually two hours.

After the treatment, the patient should rest for several minutes in a lying position but be encouraged to sit up quite soon. Resting and lying down for too long could increase *Kapha* in the head and lead to numerous signs of discomfort like giddiness, nausea, disorientation.

Some patients might need even more than one hour until they are ready to leave due to a drop in BP or dizziness.

Precautions for applying Shirodhara to traumatised patients, according to the research at Society of Friends, Berlin:

The patient should be seen and diagnosed well some time in advance of the first application of Shirodhara. Unlike media and advertisements suggest, Shirodhara is not a wellness treatment. The application of Shirodhara is a method to connect with oneself and soothe the troubled mind and the anxious heart. To establish a pattern of positive physical and mental response, a frequent repetition of the treatment is necessary. Even relaxation needs training. The relaxation method must be repeated several times until the pattern truly manifests as a change in response and behaviour.

For traumatised patients, each time the procedure of Shirodhara is performed, it will be cautiously prolonged for around 5-15 minutes—according to the patient's reaction:

- during Shirodhara,
- immediately after,
- after one hour and
- the next day.

Close monitoring of the patient is needed to show any signs of increased stress or anxiety response during the next 24 hours.

Research studies from my colleague A.K. Sharma, Jaipur, Rajasthan and Miss Gupta show a significant drop in sleeplessness in patients. Sleeplessness can signify *Cittovega* and *Unmada* and other minor and temporary stress symptoms have been reduced.

However, the second table displays more of significant changes in patients' other factors like the inability to concentrate, mood disturbances and irritability. The research study was carried out with a standardised group of patients, all middle-aged, married and government workers with similar educational backgrounds. Compared to the trauma studies on American soldiers, where groups were heterogenic from the research study background of patients, however, more similar about the trauma the above study had a more homogenic test group as a source for research recruited.

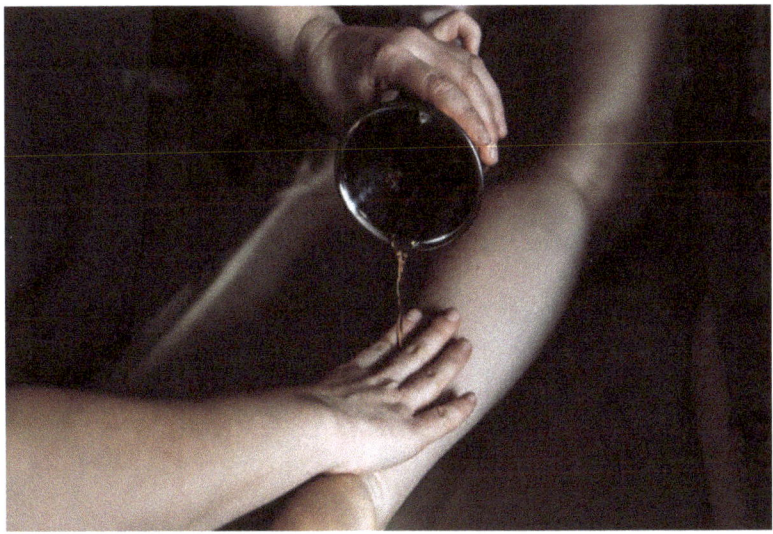

Photo: Dr Anastasia Shchedrina performing a *dhara* on the limbs
Photo credit: Natalia Smirnova, 2019

Different Techniques of Olation of the Head

- *Shiro Abhyanga*: The gentle way to begin with the introduction to relaxation is *shiro abhyanga*. Oil is gently rubbed into the hair and scalp. As it is suggested against sleeplessness and easy to apply alone without the help of a therapist, it is mainly used as a home remedy to support the effects of the other Shiro treatments.
- *Shirodhara*: A deeper level of *shiro* than shiro abhyanga (head) treatment is *shirodhara*, which penetrates the *srotas* of *rasa* and *rakta*. *Shirodhara* is a *seka*, a streaming treatment.
- *Shiro Picchu*: Instead of Shirodhara, the pouring version, a steady application of oil is applied with a cotton cloth on the forehead. It is often considered more effective, as the running oil is still a movement, therefore increasing *vataja*.

The piece of cloth is soaked in medicated oil and then fixed with a bandage.it will sit f for at least 15 minutes in position. Therefore, the bandage should be covered if the room temperature is below blood temperature.

- *Shiro Basti*: The most intense method of oil application on the head is a cylinder fixated on the skull. In most cases, the patient's hair is completely removed to achieve the best treatment results. According to the *Shastras*, this method is merely used for very severe cases of *Cittodvega*. It is widely used for Parkinson's disease.

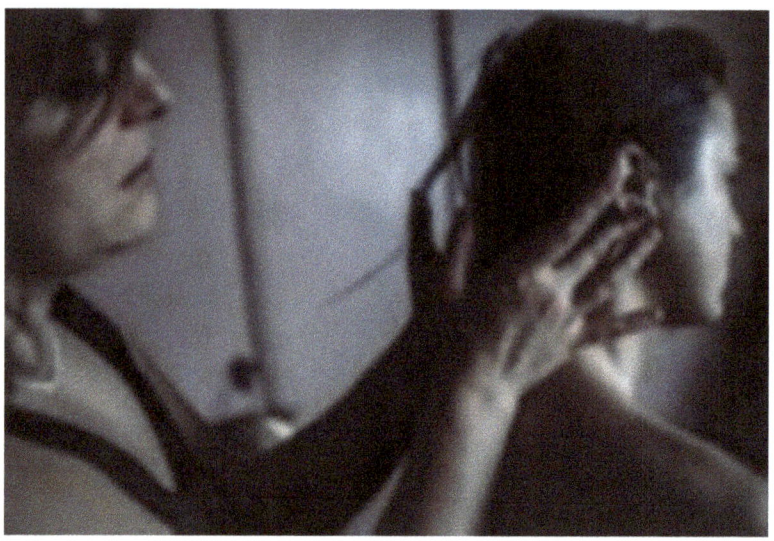

Photo: Therapist Anastasia Shchedrina prepares a patient for Shirodhara treatment with a gentle massage using Brahmi oil. Photo by the Natalia Smirnova, Society of Friends, Berlin, 2019

Looking into the different head treatment options, Shirodhara is an effective, gentle, powerful method to alter the reaction from distress in the brain. After a minimum of five to six sessions, better ten sessions, the patient's response to the method is relatively stable and predictable.

The best effects with *Shirodhara* in the treatment of Insomnia (Global Advances in Health and Medicine, published 2014) are expected when further treatments are used at the same time:

A previous *Abhyanga* treatment increases the effect of *Shirodhara*, as well as selected Herbal Therapy.

152

Still, it is to mention that besides all the factors like the nature and quality of the oil, the setting, the massage—it is the therapist, the *vaidya* or ayurvedic doctor that plays a significant role in the process of recovery. Trust and a safe space are as important as the clinical appliance of medicated oils. *Shirodhara* as just a wellness treatment method in a spa will, unfortunately, decrease the trust in the treatment in cases where there is not much hope left.

However, as mentioned earlier my research into Shirodhara for PTSD has shown results that are promising We have here for the first time methods and variations published on altering the *shirodhara* treatment in order to reduce unwanted side effects. The patient's condition is always the key to the correct application of any (ayurveda) treatment whatsoever.

Pancakarma: The Crown of Treatments

A key method, almost an entrance door to a serious change in the stress response through ayurveda medicine, is doubtlessly the *Panc Karma*. As Prof. Ram Manohar mentioned, without *Panc Karma,* no cure for the mind (for example against depression) could be successfully performed. (Private talks in Birstein, 2019)

Pancakarma is a complex treatment from India. It varies from the North to the South in medical background and the use of certain fats and oils for the treatments are different. In Northern India, ghee-based medicine is used. The South has a priority on coconut oil-based products.

Pancakarma is a group of therapies meant for radical expulsion of harmful accumulations from the body those are not eliminated through routine excretory procedures. In this way, these therapies bring the body's milieu to a normal state.

Despite regular excretion of stool, urine, sweat and other excreta in the course of life, morbid substances in cells, tissues and passages of the human body get accumulated. It is obvious that these substances have an effect on the functions of the body and a breeding ground for the development of different diseases. Such accumulations are caused both by external as well as internal factors—

Source: Possible of Modes of Action of Panca karma Therapies, 4th International Conference on Pancakarma.

(Please note, there is no differentiation on the meaning of the writing of Pancha Karma, Panchakarma, Panc Karma, Panca Karma, all mean: 5 actions, however, due to modernisation of transcriptions there are different spellings)

There are various descriptions of the multiple benefits of *Panc Karma* treatments. The explanations range from western scientific lab test-supported findings to classical texts and their interpretation.

It is important to understand that all performed therapeutic actions are according to the individual's needs and the options of the medical staff, how, what and when to perform those actions. The effect of the process is the criteria can only be seen clearly if the *Panc Karma* has been completed correctly. There is no fixed curriculum or layout that should be followed strictly. Therefore, there are many different approaches in India and even more when the treatment pattern adapts to western patients and clinicians.

However, there are three main steps to follow:

Purva karma is the first phase of increasing or moderating Agni as the preliminary procedure, Pradhana Karma is what we were performing in my clinic, basically the inner and outer olation and according to symptoms, the 5 karmas, Pachat Karma then is the time that follows, in our case we had an optional follow up for 6 weeks. .

In Europe, ayurveda has different education standards than it does have in its homeland. It does not require 10 years of studies at an ayurveda university like in most places in India, sometimes a weekend workshop is enough for someone to feel competent to start an ayurveda practice. The aspect of cultural appropriation is something to have a closer look into, the same as in yoga, as it disqualifies ayurveda on Wikipedia as pseudoscientific before the respect for it has proven the enormous healing qualities of its ancient empiric healing system.

The *Panc karma* treatment centres in Germany vary much in price and quality however, there is unfortunately no relation between price and quality. German Government regulations however, increase the safety of most places compared to the pretty much unregulated market in India. As one can see, there is a very different situation how ayurveda is studied and practiced in India and in the west.

In India:

High educational standards at Universities in several places in India

Possibly years of apprenticeships with vaidyas or in hospitals.

More safety for the patient by only same sex therapists.

But:

Generally no required laboratory testing of herbs on heavy metal pollution, pesticides, herbicides or of the preparation in total, including storage in plastic containers or recycled paper boxes.

No official and officially monitored regulations of where and how a Vaidya is allowed to practise.

No follow up by government, concerning moral or ethical conduct of the Vaidya or healer.

The current situation of ayurveda regulations in Germany.

Institutionally organised standard education as a naturopath (Heilpraktiker) is required for treating patients, however, not for being an ayurvedic massage therapist. Medical and paramedical personal is allowed to treat with less official requirements than Heilpraktiker. Heilpraktiker are allowed to diagnose and treat. Basic medical knowledge is tested by the government for naturopaths before they are allowed to open a practice.

However, the educational standards are still very low and need to be observed more closely. Particularly during the Covid Pandemic few Naturopaths overstepped the boundaries that the government had laid out. Better educational standards need to be achieved as soon as possible.

Government control and high fines in case of verified complaints. The practitioner has to keep records of the patients for 10 years.

High standard safety tests for the import of herbs and substances from outside Europe.

No educational requirement concerning ayurveda.

No regular or standard check on the qualification of the institutions that offer ayurveda studies, workshops or other.

Import restrictions of the European Union concerning herbs from Asia do not allow to use complex and proven ayurveda herbal formulas. For further information, check the laws of Novel Food, Food supplements and spices published and updated by the EU.

Drug and medical herbal safety standards are regulated for the patient's safety, leading to only a limited variety of natural medicine preparations available in the European Union (EU law-making concerning novel food, medicine and spices regulation). German laws for natural medicine are even stricter than those of the EU alone. Some ayurvedic medical preparations are illegal in German, like Septilin or Liv 52, both produced by Himalaya Herbals, as the combination of plants, minerals and animal products in one preparation is illegal in Germany despite the legality of all single substances.

Panc Karma, east and west

Generally speaking, most of the ayurvedic *Panc karma* clinics in India are of very high standard. However, travelling (no matter by foot, horse or, in modern times, airplanes, cars—) is not advisable before and after the procedure and therefore the patient flying in and out from the west is already breaking the most important rule: keeping Vata under control. Most patients arriving in India cannot fit a 5-12 weeks treatment into their tight schedule and a shorter period of time, plus the travel, does not serve the purpose of a retreat anymore.

Therefore, *Pan Karma* treatments in Europe can fill the need for the western patient—but only just. However, the benefits are they are accessible, have higher safety standards and are government-controlled. But the originality of herbal decoctions, medicine preparations and personal intensive care plus the long-time treatments are limiting the desired effect. Trauma-sensitive practitioners are hard to find. Complex psychiatric issues like PTSD treatments, like Unmada and Cittodvega are not part of their education, neither in the west nor in the east.

What can we expect from a Panc Karma in general?

As a Panc Karma can be performed for the person of ill health, due to its adaptability, it can be used for prevention as well.

Not only physical ailments are improving, restorative functions are stabilised, the sense organs are cleared and so important for patients with traumatic experience, the mind gets calm and pacified, further we saw a decline of use of recreational drugs, cigarettes and alcohol that lasted for more than 6 months minimum, a repetition was often required until all the self-harming behaviour was eradicated.

Particularly, our patients that struggled with multi morbidity and poly toxic problems reported that they had no withdrawal symptoms whatsoever no withdrawal means, no craving to get rid of the withdrawal. We could help without judging, lecturing or making the patient feel guilty or ashamed.

We used Panc Karma in many classical ways to enhance fertility, sexual vigour and stamina. So it is a vital part of our fertility treatments. The general improvement of physical strength is having a positive impact on victims of trauma that felt nervous and frail. Physical strength induces a feeling of being safe.

A short overview of Panc Karma treatment options differing from Vata, Kapha or Pitta conditions, simplified here, the treatments of the 5 karmas (Panc karma) are chosen carefully. Wrong choices can lead to harmful increasing of previous symptoms or to the appearance of new symptoms. Symptoms of a failed Panc Karma are difficult to treat. Those symptoms are mostly: strong joint pain like rheumatoid pain, fever, chronic headaches, changes in digestion, flare up of skin diseases, fever and many more. In my clinic, we have been treating a number of patients coming from Panc Karmas in Germany who suffered from new and bad symptoms. characterised by Ama.

reating Vata symptoms is mostly the start of any Panc Karma treatment .Procedures like *Vamana* (emesis) are necessary; for instance, if there is Kapha blocking the sinus, the lungs or any other space, but it can also reduce Pitta from the stomach region and free the diaphragm. A diagnose of the produce of vamana is taken in consideration for further treatments. Bastis (herbal enema) are used to treat Vata in the intestine; however, there is a differentiation made between oil and watery enemas for each condition.

Nasya is used for mental disorders as well as for congestions of the orifices of the head. Herbal decoctions for evacuation through the intestine are also used for Vata conditions, while *Raktamokshana* (bloodletting) is primarily used to control Pitta. However, this is basically just the start. Snehana, the inner and out olation, will be performed, steam baths and saunas, sandbags, *Pizhili* (stamps soaked in hot medicated oil or milk) and other treatments like *Abhyanga*, *Shirodhara* in the right amount and for the right condition are orchestrated by the ayurveda therapist.

An interesting fact in *Panc Karma* is that on the first glimpse, it seems to be only a physical treatment procedure. There is no counselling, no western approved psychological therapy program included. Besides a short introductory anamnestic talk with the patient, there is no talking at all. Therapists enrol all the procedures, specifically trained for the specific treatments. As certain procedures require more strength and compassion, well-trained staff is a key to a successful outcome.

Besides the physical treatment of oil massages, water applications, sand bags, pouring oil, rubbing, steaming mental issues are well addressed under

Panc Karma. This is very different to western physical therapy which uses hot sand, deep tissue massage, heat, cold etc as well however, one would not necessarily advise patients suffering from Unmada/Cittodveda, PTSD etc. to see a physiotherapist.

Clinical trials show nevertheless a reduction of depression, sleeplessness and anxiety. Research gate and pubmed are well known platforms for scientific exchange of clinical trials in the scientific world according to my own observation I would always suggest a Panc Karma treatment for people suffering from PTSD symptoms, as Prof. Ram Manohar has suggested.

As much I myself was surprised in the beginning, the more treatments I could perform, the more I am now convinced over the importance for this particular treatment in case of Unmada/Cittodvega.

Treatment approaches to Trauma:

Pranayama, Panc Karma and *Shirodhara*—ways *to* self-regulation and recovery

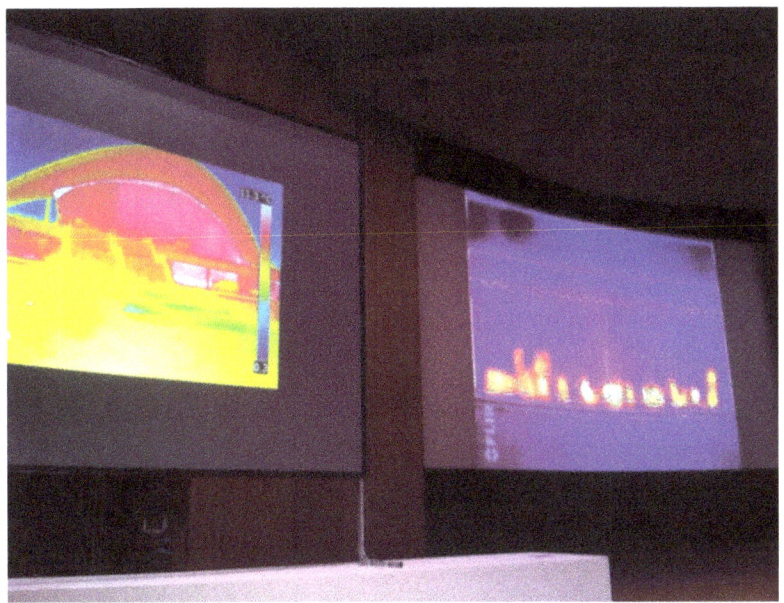

Photo:, the author. A project during the exhibition and research project: Anthropozaen, curated by Ashkan Sepahvand, Berlin, in: Haus der Kulturen der Welt (house of the world cultures) 2010; the author was leading a *pranayama*—intro while the participants were photographed with an infrared camera. The picture above displays the brightness of all bodies (on the right) after the session. The general body temperature was increased between 0.5-1 degrees Celsius during breathing. It had even slightly changed the room temperature, which can be seen in the slightly pink areas above the individual's bright light fields

Pranayama: The Yogic Breathing

The practice of pranayama as a tool of excellence for treatment is widely underestimated. However, the regular practice only is what leads to recovery and healing. These days a growing number of modern breathing techniques like psychedelic breathwork, holotrophic breathing are coming up that persuade the practitioner with hallucinations, DMT-like experiences and other strong experiences.

For pranayama as for all healing in the context of yoga and ayurveda, we actually focus on practice and avoid single strong events. Changes have to be embedded in subtle experiences for recovery, peak experiences are often adding to stress. Even this stress is considered as positive stress first, the same biochemical release of stress hormones happens, but the perception is different. In my experiences, continuity and regular regimen are the tools that lead to positive changes on all the fields of the patient's life and circumstances on their way to recovery.

As much as everyone is conscious that we are breathing, little is known about the science of altering the breath. First, one has to discover the authentical breath that each individual owns. From there, the observation into alternation starts like an adventure. The breath-hold is a key to understand the response to traumatic experiences and, surprisingly, seems to be a crucial tool in the way of recovery.

When a victim is exposed to a vital threat (including abusive devaluating language although the person will not die physically by strong words), the breath flow alters and can even stop. The breath gets shallow, the sensitive mucus tissue in the nose shrinks if the inhalation gets sharp. Oxygenation and carbon dioxide levels in the blood are low.

Treatment with Yogic Breathing

The Deep Practice towards Recovery, Self—Control, Arousal Management and Self-Esteem

The empirical knowledge in which *pranayama* techniques have been used for 35 years on my patients in Berlin explains the key tool for: The ayurveda/yoga Treatment of *Unmada/Cittovega* and Psychological Trauma. A dedicated self-practice is needed to get trained these techniques, for the therapist as for the patient.

Although the primary treatment approach to be analysed and presented in this book is clearly is the science of ayurveda—the combination with healing methods from *Patanjali* Yoga and *Gheranda Samhita* have significantly impacted the overall recovery and resilience of the patients.

Most of the beneficial ayurveda treatments depend on a trained therapist who applies oil, massages or chooses herbs. Knowledge and education in the field are needed. *Pranayama,* after a good introduction, can be performed alone at home at any time and is free of costs.

The combination of ayurveda's *ahara/vihara* (lifestyle and food management), plus the daily practice of *pranayama* have been more efficient in my research than the ayurveda treatments alone (including herbs and lifestyle management, as well as the application of medicated oil in *Abhyanga* or *Shirodhara* treatments) within the therapeutic setting. Part of it was definitely the time/ money issue with the majority of patients, as ayurveda requires both.

Using *pranayama* as part of the therapy plan, the therapist can offer a supportive treatment that:

- Does not cost anything,
- the patient does not have to go anywhere,
- the patient will feel the soothing and focusing results immediately,
- the treatment effect intensifies with practice,
- Scientific evidence is acquired by measuring the heartbeat rate, pulse, breath volume.

(For the studies at Society of Friends, Berlin, the following tools were at use: free heartbeat rate, the app for iPhone, Omron digital blood pressure monitor with app stored information, Pulse Oximeter and most patients actually owned an apple watch which displays most of the needed functional parameters)

Some of my traumatised patients have been successfully and solely relying on *pranayama* for their recovery, yet embedded in a self-responsible lifestyle and nutrition regime which often followed naturally and did not have to be reinforced. The case study of Kabir will illuminate the tremendous power of *pranayama* and meditation. *Pranayama* can be a foundation for meditation but it is a method in itself.

Meditation is generally not advisable for patients with *Unmada/Cittovega* or other mental or psychological disturbances. However, it is often taught for patients with stress, burn-out or other symptoms of Unmada/Cittodvega. Please note that meditation, as it is merely taught in the west, is not identical with the meditation as *Dhyana* according to *Patanjali Yoga*.

It is simply not possible for an agitated the patient to suddenly sit quietly while being emotionally overwhelmed. The result of even a brave attempt towards meditation is often re another experience of dissociation from the HERE and NOW.

As a patient told me: "The insight into the trauma memory and re-experiencing of fear was triggered by being told to sit still with closed eyes—when anxiety and contents of trauma were displayed again and again. All the suffering came back, crushing me, burying me and taking away all that I had achieved." (Patient W., 2019)

Pranayama can be a way to control emotions by pacifying the physical response. It teaches the patient awareness of the breath and its alterations under stressful circumstances long before the patient fully experiences the stress. By controlling the breath, the arousal can be settled faster before the whole cascade of panic, freezing, increase in heartbeat rate, cold sweat, dry mouth, etcetera, appears. The breathwork can be introduced as a primary technique in the treatment process or taught during unique ayurveda treatments like *abhyanga* or *shirodhara*.

The numerous benefits of treating emotional trauma and *pranayama* practice are explained in great detail. Any therapist can follow these guidelines easily yet should acquire the knowledge of practical appliances through intense self-practice first.

After years of inefficient use and even adverse effects during *pranayama,* we at Society of Friends, Berlin, realised that a categorisation system is needed for the best treatment choices. From the years of experience, we could start defining patterns for treatments. The foundation for those therapeutic choices has to be a profound knowledge of the *doshas* and the *gunas.* From these ayurveda patterns, exploration can gradually start into the unknown of the patient's minds and memories.

Once the therapist is familiar with the possible reactions on a *dosha/guna* level and the bio-physical level during and after each *pranayama* technique, an adaption and fine-tuning the practice for each individual patient is possible. There might be days where there is progress, all seems to go smooth and recovery is close—until a sound, a smell, tears away the curtain of dissociation and the patient stares again into the traumatic experience. Just as if nothing had been achieved in the weeks before.

In such cases, the therapist should know different options on how to perform each *pranayama* technique in subtle variations according to the needs, alter the breath counts or even the methods.

My case studies on hundreds of patients treated with the combination of ayurveda and pranayama have convinced me to propose the combination of ayurveda and yoga, particularly *pranayama*. In the treatment of trauma. Even when the patient feels lost again, with a pleasure that leads to pain again—the opportunity to find the way back into relaxation and increased positive self—

awareness remains. Advanced breathing methods are a straightforward way to recover and even better with a selection of herbs or massage, shirodhara or other ayurveda treatments like *Panc Karma.*

Effects of therapy with *Pranayama* at Society of Friends, Berlin, 2020 (research lay out and statistics by the author)

Patients Observed have been about 250 patients over a time of 10 years	General feeling after 1 week of practice on a scale from 1 to 10 improvement	After 5 weeks	After 6 months	1 year	Backdrop by forgetting about the practice
Childhood trauma, abuse starting from early age	7	3	8	5	Generally after 6 months
Sexual insult As adult	6	3	8	6	Mostly after 1 year
War crime, refugees	4	6	7	9	90 percent were continuing the practice
Victim of physical assault, domestic violence Terror attacks (in general not more than 1—2 incidents)	3	6	7	9	90 percent were continuing the practice

The chart displays a significant diversity in responses to the practice according to the cause of the psychological trauma. However, the chart does not display overlapping traumatic injuries in the same individual. Often patients who suffered from childhood abuse tend to expose themselves unwantedly to further traumatising situations. Their boundaries are weakly defined.

Several patients who had a bad start in life are more likely to become victims of domestic violence, which is the case for men and women equally (not in total numbers). Women are more likely to seek help and receive support (mainly as they care for minors), unlike men who got involved in domestic violence. Men as victims of domestic violence seldomly call the police for support. In particular, male POCs (People of Colour) in the US and other countries fear rather discrimination than hoping to receive support.

The backdrop in practice displays a difference between people who became victims once and continued staying in problematic relationships, abusive and devaluating workplaces or other retraumatising conditions. Workplaces can be traumatising per se: like fire brigades, first aid responder, hospiz workers, psychiatric nurses and so many more. These patients did often not continue the practice by heart. But people, who escaped war, crimes or violent domestic attacks were more likely to continue the practice regularly and therefore harvested the full benefits of the technique.

For later patients, the change in life's circumstances by leaving the threatening place made a difference. Many of those patients with refugee backgrounds originated from Palestine or were Palestinians from Syria or Iraq. For them and their children, having arrived in Germany and becoming a German passport holder has made a drastic positive change in their life's perspective. The practice of *pranayama* was a constant reminder of a safe place, a "home away from home," an anchor.

A great number of patients who suffered sexual assault were able to start new intimate relationships. They frequently reported feeling uncomfortable introducing their new partners to their painful past. They usually reached out for another practice class to get back on track whenever a relationship had ended. Patients exposed to domestic violence or terror attacks with only one incident were more likely to continue the practice without longer interruptions.

Patients who experienced a childhood of abuse, severe neglect or even sexual assault were more likely to be a bit "overly enthusiastic" initially. Those patients often tried to please the therapist in order to be liked. "To be likeable" can give a false sense of security, but it is manipulative and not an honest start for a profound change. When the therapist is to "like" the patient, the expectation is that, that the therapist would not confront the patient with anything unpleasant.

(" Everything the therapist told me I already knew, but then she wanted to speak about all the things I don' t want to speak about, she is not good, I don't like her, she is not nice to me", Patient D, 2021.)

This behaviour is rooted in avoidance. The overly adapted child with great marks in school, the cleanliest housewife, the flawless teenager fit into the

164

category of overly adapted people. However, the second column shows a drastic drop in the overall experienced improvement. Here, the patients start to complain about that "nothing that the therapist does is working" at this phase. Most of these patients have not been practicing regularly, but they narcissistically, pitta-driven, tend to blame the therapist: "it is their fault."

These patients are unaware of their emotional or dosha structure that lead to avoidance physically or mentally challenging practices. The sounds of heavy breath or the smell of sweat are difficult to handle for some people as of their triggering aspects, which must be considered as problematic but avoidable.

The above experiences lead to the new individualised *pranayama* system for the treatment of Unmada/Cittodvega or PTSD and other. *dosha* and *guna* aspects should always be considered as they are the keys to customise the program and preferably include ayurveda treatments.

Examples of Variations of Pranayama for treatments:

Pranayama is a technique of directing the breath. Its science is vast and modern findings on breathing, breath control, breath hold, ice swimming, freediving and many more are just coming up. However, they all shed a fascinating light on breathing. The recent book of James Nestor is an easy-to-read book which allows the reader to dive deep into the history of different breathing techniques, the influence of our food choices, our health in connection with our breathing as a stress reduction method or, in case of obstructed airways, wrong breathing as a significant stress increasing factor.

Mostly, all modern scientists agree that we are breathing too much, too shallow. We are breathing with open mouths at night and even very often during the day. Nose breathing alone can change the heartbeat rate and the stress level, like one can observe in simple apps on watches or phones as HRV, heart rate variability.

Teaching breathing allows the therapist to adapt the breath frequency, depth, speed of inhalation as for exhalation to the individual patients. pranayama gives great freedom to the therapist to experiment, observe, challenge, change, adapt, force, let go, everything is possible and all alterations can be corrected, changed, intensified within seconds—

Yet the structure of the breathing mode is essential. Using ayurveda's diagnostic tools to verify the choices of the alterations made.

The following variations can be applied:

- the time of inhalation can be shortened
- the time of inhalation can be lengthened-
- the time of exhalation could be shortened
- the time of exhalation can be lengthened
- the pause after inhalation can be lengthened
- the pause after inhalation can be shortened
- the pause after exhalation can be lengthened
- the pause after exhalation can be shortened
- no pause after inhalation
- no pause after exhalation
- long breath hold empty lung
- long breath hold full lung
- movements while breathing
- physical stillness while breathing
- the breath flows into the side chest
- the breath flows into the back chest
- the breath flows into the front chest
- the breath flows into the belly
- the breath flows into the kidneys
- application of ice cubes or cold water on the points of the mammalian dive reflex points
- patients are allowed to get loud
- patients can become so subtle that the breath is almost unheard
- patients can practice it while walking or swimming, but never unattended (not while diving!)
- patients can be quiet or extra loud after the training
- Combining the pranayama with water: use free-diving skills like a wet cloth on the face to control the heartbeat rate. Experiment: A bowl filled with ice water so that the face can dive in is a tremendous positive challenge for some people.

In my eyes, any breathwork and any breathing teaching that changes the flow, the frequency, the intensity, the depth, the direction, the mode for short terms, longer terms, intervals of the patient's breath requires skills that one can only achieve by long term and honest self-practice.

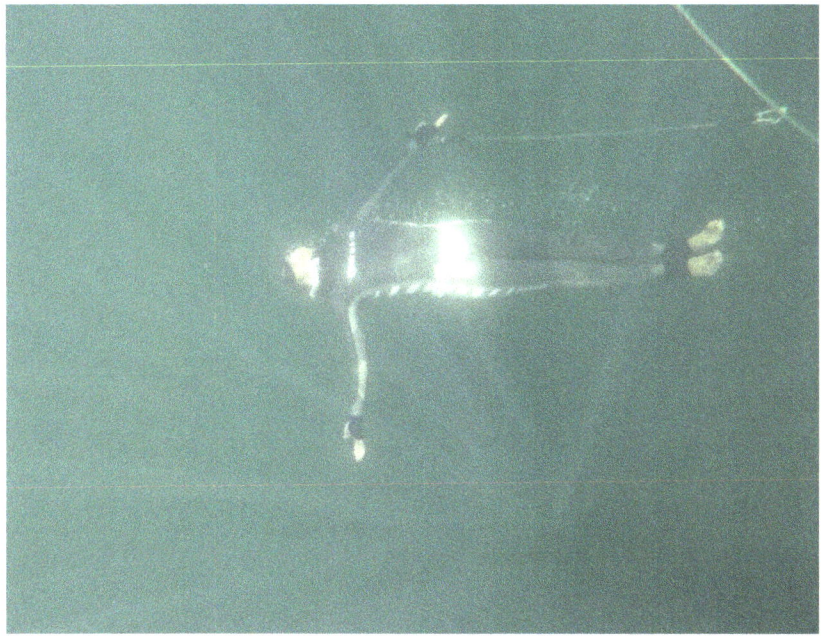

Photocredit: Jessica Schäfer, onebreathme

The author, freediving 20m, Germany 2022, August, Gräbendorfer See

The Study of the Self: Skill Training in Self-Care and Self-Acceptance
The breath that moves inside you

In my experience, it is an absolute must that the therapist is having a profound self-practice, as I was able to observe dozens of students working with hundreds of patients under my guidance. The inexperienced students frequently had to interrupt the session and ask for help, they reported more sleep disturbances, even anxiety issues in the first weeks after working with patients. These symptoms did not occur if working with experienced breathing teachers or therapists with a proper self-practice. They, in fact, reported an increase of their overall wellbeing, even after long days of breath therapy.

The therapist explains how the breathing class will be structured, performed (what style: breath hold, cathartic breathing, silence—), what to expect (a journey of self-observation, looking into comfort and discomfort), what hindrances could occur (light-headedness, tightness in the chest), when it will end (this is maybe the most important bit) in clear and simple words. The therapist should be to able to precisely perform the different *pranayama* methods themself.

The active breathing methods should be studied by heart and a daily practice is necessary to achieve the benefit of any *pranayama* technique. Without the therapist's self-experience of *pranayama*, they can hardly be convincing. As it is truly a life-saving key tool, it is taken to be as seriously as any method in psychology or psychiatry.

However, like the practice of meditation, the effect of *pranayama* is not lasting, if not routinely done. ("OK, I meditated now, I finished the *pranayama*, what s next?" patient D,2020)

Although the experience of an immediate change occasionally happens, it is only the regular and dedicated practice with an open mind and heart, without expectations or excuses that *pranayama* practice will present long-lasting changes.

Suggestions for deepening the practice of Pranayama

The therapist can advise the patients to write a daily *pranayama* experience diary, to make notes about their experiences, on and off the mat and even write down their observed excuses for avoiding the practice, is an excellent help to stick—to—the—plan, even in difficult times. Looking back after some time is often an eye opening how much progress has actually been achieved.

Advise for therapists and students:

Start writing your own a *pranayama* journal if you are not already doing so. It is important to understand one's own mindset and the structure of one's own excuses and patterns of avoidance. Working with U*nmada/Cittodvega* and psychological trauma needs empathy and practical skills that only can be developed by self-experience.

How to Introduce the Patient to *Pranayama*: Making the Right Choice of Practice

Treatment with Breathing: The Deep Practice Towards Recovery, Self-Control, Arousal Management and Self Esteem

The Setting for the safe-space

Pranayama can be practiced literally anywhere and in any position. To start with a new patient, it is advisable to find a comfortable position for both, the patient and the therapist.

For the first sessions, the therapist can preferably offer a comfortably bolstered chair to sit on. One could also use a couple of pillows, bolsters, cushions or other support to allow the patient to sit as cosy and comfortable as possible. Practicing *pranayama* in a wheelchair or bedbound is not a problem, which makes it a rare method in the field of practiced exercises that can be done by anyone, anywhere, under any circumstances.

Only patients who are already familiar and truly comfortable sitting on the floor or a yoga mat can be asked to sit on the floor for more than 15 minutes. A firm blanket provided to sit on is helpful to provide a more relaxed setting when choosing the floor. Even just a firmly folded blanket alters the response of the parasympathetic nervous system in a seated position, and, as much as the person feels comfortable, they will be able to follow the instructions by not being distracted by unnecessary discomfort.

Psychologically traumatised patients have a fight-or-flight response-reaction if Vata is dominating, an anger-aggression response if pitta-dominated and dissociation-freeze response if Kapha-dominated if anything that feels wrong along the way and triggers the memory of the traumatic experience. A wrong setting can lead to their dosha /guna dominated stress response.

Under these circumstances, the therapist has not achieved any change for the better but has created a strong feeling of aversion towards the therapy. It often takes quite some time to re-establish a connection between the therapist and the patient once the patient felt insecure or overwhelmed during the treatment.

The Safe Space

The therapist creates a safe space by reducing, but not eliminating, outside sounds and disturbances during the treatment time. In my years of working with traumatised patients at my clinic, Society of Friends, a silenced treatment room had frequently even increased the onset of a panic reactions. Any sudden sound or disturbance into the silence was experienced intensified.

The slightest even familiar sound coming from outside and breaking into the silence, like road noises, people talking, a telephone ringing in the kitchen had created more mental disturbances than an open window in the summer where the patient is exposed to a lullaby of sounds that are not connected to them and they will simply not react and even forget them.

Another important note: the patients need to be ensured that everything is confidential, unless they give their permission to cooperate with other therapists or speak to partners or relatives. In Germany, the rules for therapists concerning private data are very strict and indecency can lead to fines and even imprisonment.

The safe space should include the agreement to safe words. The patient can name a particular word that interrupts the session when it gets too uncomfortable.

Trust between two parties needs time to grow. All therapeutic settings should respect time as an essential part of the treatment. One cannot rush someone into trust.

Awareness in speech is important. Phrases like: You can do it if you really want, try harder, I told you that should do this, can trigger previous and often abusive experiences.

Creating a Dialogue

Creating a dialogue means to learn about the patient on different layers than just the verbal exchange can bring. The dialogue includes, touch (of the pulse), listening to the breath, observing the posture, finding blind spots in the previous examination and from there only decide about treatment options. It is more than talking and listening and much more subtle and connecting than a medical anamnesis.

Understanding body language, facial expressions, even the change of smell of the patient's sweat is an art that needs time and practice to be developed. The patient is in an alert and stressed situation when starting with a new environment, a new therapist or just a new technique. Therefore, even the body language, facial expression and relaxation of the therapist themselves their own breathing patterns are a big part of the dialogue. It is essential to explore how much physical distance is necessary between the patient and the therapist (or if there are more patients, between all of them in the group) and create a proper setting in the room.

Patients from different cultural backgrounds feel differently about distance. A reasonable comfortable distance for a Japanese person may be awkward for a Brazilian, who might feel rejected by the space a Japanese may need to bend forward for a formal greeting. Clinical studies at Society of Friends, Berlin, international programs for the European Union discovered a lot of cultural differences when it comes to working distance in yoga therapy*.

Every person has different feelings, needs and emotions towards distance and space and children. As general advice, the therapist should sit down first to decide where to place themself relative to the therapist.

For the *Vata* personality in *Vkrit* there is the famous saying: the person needs so much space around them that then they feel lonely inside the space.

Choosing the right location for the patient is not difficult if the therapist simply asks the patient. There had been often an unnecessary confusion of my students towards the therapeutic settings and surprisingly none of them thought of the option to ask the patient. Therapists often live under the threat that if they ask they might lose their credibility. Patients experience the question mostly in a different way: someone asks how I am, what I prefer, how I feel.

As this can be healing in itself, it can also trigger. The therapist therefore cannot have a ready-made, over-all working check list but has to learn to react quickly to different reactions of the patients. this again needs a lot of experience, preferably under supervision. I am asking here for better education standards in *pranayama*, ayurveda and complementary medicine in Europe and elsewhere. Even though, with growing experience, patients might answer: "I don't care," the therapist should offer different options.

It is possible to try several options in the beginning to feel the differences and only then make a choice, it is for the sitting as well as for the breathing and even for the ayurveda treatments While observing the patient's reactions, the therapist can most likely find out where and how the patient feels comfortable or uncomfortable, both important information—whether in front of the door, facing a window or close to the wall should be options offered and given a try. The patient usually appreciates this subtle inquiry and might even experience a feeling of valuation towards their needs.

The therapist should avoid strong smells of perfumes, washing detergent, incense or body products as traumatic as well as other memories are attached to smell. The sense of smell is the first that appears in humans after birth and the last to go in death. It is the most sensitive sensor for the detection of shelter and danger. The sense of smell often triggers memories. The less the therapist is leaving a trace of scent, the better!

Introducing Care and Comfort

The therapist should be able to create a feeling of security, care and comfort at all times. The safe space is the important space where change can only happen.

Some patients enjoy the offer of tea, water, juice and a short conversation about topics other than the psychological trauma or how they feel today. The question about today might bring back the memory of unwanted scenes as an aftermath of trauma. They might still be living in a narcissistic relationship, been gaslighted or other sad circumstances that throw a shadow over the moment in which they are right now, the moment of starting the practice to open the doors for new experiences.

So comforting the patient, looking after them kindly without being invasive is important. The patient needs the feeling of a new beginning in a safe environment. Ayurveda and yoga can provide this by their very nature of treatment.

Safety First

During the *pranayama* setting the therapist should allow the patient to sit with open eyes. There is no need to close the eyes to experience *pranayama*. The same rule is for all Yoga Asana practice valid. Eyes closed can cause emotional flareups as the patient loses immediately contact with what's around them. When they finally relax, the eyes will start flittering, slowly close-open until they finally might close without having had the intention. It can be used as an indicator of the progress of overall relaxation.

The safe space includes the surrounding during treatment. Checking how the patient feels about blinds in front of the window can be important as it can differ between people according to their experiences. Blinds can feel like a protective shield from the outside world or like a threat as they feel trapped. For some people, privacy is essential and they will not relax until it is clear they are not seen. The opposite reaction could be the case for other patients: no one can look into the room, no one could come for help!

The therapist cannot know everything but can always ask! Asking is an excellent way to show that the therapist is connected to the patient and cares about them.

Asking the Patient: "How are you today?"

It is advisable to avoid the question at the beginning of the class. My studies on patients at Society of Friends, Berlin, showed that the question often led to long and distracting conversations. These conversations mainly served the purpose to avoid relaxation and to escape even positive effects during and after *pranayama*. The pleasure avoidance or pleasure resistance pattern is a typical pattern that can be seen in the majority of traumatised patients. Avoiding pleasurable moments on all levels, like on desire, sexual pleasure, eating and other is rooted in the feelings of guilt and shame.

During extended monologues form the patients the verbal distraction of the therapist easily leads to confusing instructions later on. Self-sabotaging behaviour can be seen as an attempt by the victim to avoid pleasure during treatment. Therefore, the therapist should avoid asking the patient about today's feelings, rather understand by observing body language, breathing patterns, focus and other signs of being emotionally stressed or relaxed at the time of the treatment.

Therapy and treatment days are usually days when patients might face unwanted memories and feelings again, particularly when the treatment with *pranayama* is new to them. Asking questions about how they feel after *pranayama* could be immensely helpful as the patient might realise and incorporate the difference they felt before and after.

Questionnaire and Diaries: A Practical Guide to *Pranayama* as Part of a Holistic Healing Plan for PTSD

How to begin:

- take a moment to observe the involuntary breathing pattern of the patient,
- Ask the patient to observe their breathing themselves first, comment on it, describe it and give simple feedback.

Questions like:

- how would you describe the flow of your breath?
- Is it moving inside you?
- Where do you feel it the most?
- Can you direct it to the areas where you feel it less?
- How does the breath feel inside you?
- how does the breath move inside you, are there restrictions, currents, does it make you cough?
- Do you feel an increase of heat in some areas?
- Do you feel getting colder in some areas?
- Do you feel an increase of any emotion?
- Do you feel a decrease in Stress, heartbeat?
- Do you feel relaxed?
- Do you want to stop?
- Do you want to continue?

It is helpful to ask every question separately as clusters of questions or questions that of the yes/no in one question can be confusing after experiencing something new.

Imagine a water scale: subtle as you move the little bubble in the water to find equilibrium, like this, the treatment with breath can restore balance. No force, no good intention, no feeling of achieving a goal will help. Only practice.

Keeping a diary of the patient's experiences is a must for the therapist. Filling in name, date, practitioner (if there are many) and any information that goes with it:

- Have they eaten before class, earlier or later?
- Have they drank coffee or alcohol recently? Have they consumed drugs—prescribed or recreational?
- Is the patient behaving respectfully or ignoring the instructions?

- Does the patient have pain? Use a scale from 1-10
- Are they in a good or bad mood?
- what is the dominant emotion?
- How do they feel?
- Have they slept well? Hardly? Badly? Dreams?
- Has the patient practiced on their own?

The therapist should write comments about all these topics for themself. The therapist's mood and stress factors influence the work with the patient. This is particularly true if the therapist sees similarities to own narratives coming up through the patients' experienced trauma.

A differentiation of responses to traumatic injuries according to the _doshas_
First stage: _Vata_
Concepts of controlling _Vata_ and reducing its symptoms of insecurity, distractedness, anxiety and flight response with _Pranayama_.

The therapist should be aware of the nature of the constant changes of _Vata_. It is easy to be disappointed when the patient excessively talks or is distracted even by minor things. The therapist should be aware that the patient is not doing this intentionally, but that this is the survival strategy to block unwanted or unfamiliar emotions. As _Vata_ is fuelling _Pitta_ and _Kapha_, one should keep in mind the _Prakriti_ and the _Vikriti_ to understand the nature of changes and the consequences more predictably.

The table below displays common reactions towards therapeutic _pranayama_ and results from hundreds of hours of study at Society of Friends, Berlin.

175

Vata-Vata	Light-headedness	Interrupting the session by constant talking, reporting different physical symptoms like nausea, dizziness, urge to urinate, cough or sneeze
Vata Pitta	Easily upset and uncomfortable, irritable	Interrupting the session by being upset, having to leave for more important things
Vata Kapha	Bored	Interrupting the session by getting tired

Nadi Shodhana

Variations according to symptoms of *Unmada/Cittovega* and Psychological Trauma.

The therapist can start the program with creating awareness, asking:

Which is the nostril that is more active at this very moment?

As the nostril activity changes almost every two hours, one can start with the subtle sensual experience of feeling length and shortening in the body according to the nostril activity. One can feel stress or relaxation just by observing the breath flow through the nostrils and trying to alter this sensation.

If it is the left nostril, the person might already be responding to the calmness of the setting and is at Vagus nerve activity. If it is the right nostril, the patient should stay some moments in simple observation. For more experienced patients, as the nostril's activity changes over the day, do not over-interpret the side information. The patient can then lie down on the side of the blocked nostril.

Direct questions guide the patient's awareness: which side of the body feels shorter? Feels longer, lighter, congested? Almost all patients with at least some compliance will be able to tell that the body feels longer on the side of the open nostril. Even if inexperienced in these methods, the patient will feel that the side of the blocked nostril feels dull, short and not soft, while the other side is more prolonged, lighter, brighter and more open.

Interesting facts to catch the attention: the therapist asks the patient to make a fist on the side with reduced breathing sensation: the blocked nostril will open.

Method:

Directing the breath from side to side. Beginning with:

- Placing index and the middle finger of the right hand on the forehead, then closing the left nostril with the ring finger and the right nostril with the thumb. The patient might experience a stressful feeling during inhalation of the blocked nostril and might even feel a slight panic just by trying to inhale.
- Creating awareness: tell the patient that it is just their finger blocking a nostril and the finger can be removed anytime without asking. They have to be assured sometimes that they are not choking.
- create a feeling of safety and empowerment.
- Slowly tell to open the one nostril, then to change sides.
- Introduce the patient carefully to a gentle and subtle breathing method. Traumatised patients tend to inhale sharply through the nose if they cannot inhale with ease, which leads to swelling of the nostril's inner lining and more blockage.

Now starting the *Nadi Shodhana* (alternating nostril breathing):

- Exhale through the right nostril, closing the left.
- Inhale through the right nostril.
- Exhale through the left nostril, closing the right.
- Inhale through the left nostril.
- Continue.

Once the breathing is directed to the other nostril, the therapist should again ask how the body feels on the same side and then how it feels on the other side. If the patient feels comfortable, the therapist can challenge them by extending the breathing phases as the length or the stops between breaths.

Introducing the Magic of Numbers: Counting

Box breathing is the simplest way to slowly adapt to a new practice. The therapist has to keep in mind that every new practice is a challenge for a traumatised patient:

Inhale while counting slowly, silently until five,

- Hold the breath counting until five.
- Exhale, counting until five.
- Hold the breath, counting until 5.
- The therapist can count slowly for the patient to make sure that they are still with the practice and not wandering off internally. Introducing counting with the fingers or using a mal can be helpful. Different tasks for the patient during breathing tasks can help the therapist to make clear observations.

For advanced students, the breathing pattern can become more flexible and even challenging:

- Exhaling, count until six.
- Holding the breath for four.
- Inhaling on four.
- Holding for four.

Or

- Exhaling on eight.
- Holding for four.
- Inhaling on six.
- Holding for four.

Or

Strong challenge:

- Inhale on 4.
- Hold on 6.
- Exhale on 6.
- Hold on 8.

There are innumerable options, just ensuring that the exhalation phase is the longest, the breath-hold stage is not getting too long and the patient is feeling comfortable.

It is important to offer a small challenge in the beginning to gain trust. The patient needs to feel that, in the presence of the therapists, they can explore something new and extend their limits. The feeling of relief after each class and then increasing the challenge can be a joyful experience. If the patient is advanced and feels secure and safe with the therapist, they can be asked to direct the breath evenly through both nostrils without closing a nostril.

It is crucial that no sound is heard of the moving breath.

The breath should flow subtle and refined.

The Subtle Breath, the Shallow Breath and the *Bandhas*

A subtle, fine breath is not at all a shallow breath. Instead, the quiet, subtle breath is a long, fine and gently filling or emptying breath that connects all three diaphragms. A shallow breath is considered a breath that results in over-breathing as only the tips of the lungs get air. The more parts of the lungs where more oxygenation happens are the bottom of the lungs. During the peak of the Corona pandemic we also saw that the actually the back of the lung allows more gas exchange, as patients were placed in hospitals in prone position.

The first diaphragm: in fact, the pelvic floor is considered to be the first diaphragm, where the breathing activity originates from. Without any force on the pelvic floor, just by the nature of the directed subtle breath, the pelvic floor will be lifted naturally and effortless during inhalation.

The second diaphragm: a gentle feeling of connection between the lower abdomen and the pelvic floor, the back side of the body and an opening of the chest can be felt. However, as our breathing muscles lack training and getting increasingly tight just by aging, The middle diaphragmatic breathing skill can cause a feeling of constriction.

With professional guidance the feeling will subside as the muscles relax and the widened chest allows free movement of all breathing muscles and inner chest organs as well as free movement of all joints that are rarely used in daily life: the joints that connect the ribs with the chest bone.

The third diaphragm: it is located in the centre of the throat. Naturally, the patient will perform a gentle *jalandhara bandha,* which is a slight and mild lock or restriction of the breath flow over the glottis which can be heard as a gentle sound like wind pipe.

The second centre of the diaphragms is called *uddhiyana bandha and* the first centre of diaphragms, the pelvic floor, is named *moola bandha*. The all experience a subtle pull towards the centre and create an immediate feeling of inner core stability. Core strength drills, like practiced in Pilates, are very different from the subtle inner stability created through the inner breath.

However, in the beginning of the practice, the increasing inner strength can be misinterpreted by the patient as restriction. The side chest muscles are stretched, the paraspinal muscles are lengthened. In case this has not been done in a long time, it can create a feeling of discomfort, tightness and locked-in sensation. The patient should be helped to relax and guided through an almost fluid movement of the breath with no force and not trying to achieve anything.

The patient should be carefully guided through the deep relaxation experience and encourage them to take some involuntary breaths to ease the control mode. In all cases, the patient will need a moment after the intense breathing experience until they open their eyes and reach out for eye contact.

In my experience, I would advise not to interrupt the slow path of coming back. Intense breathing is a deep meditative inner experience and so the way to move into the breathing, to be in the breathing and to come out of the breathing experience should be a smooth and gentle transition where all 3 parts are equally practiced.

In the beginning of breathing therapy, the therapist should be guiding only a few breathing rounds. Three to five rounds of breathing are usually enough for absolute beginners. The patient should feel that they could integrate the breathing as daily life practice where they won't do anything wrong.

Kumbhaka and *Rechaka*, meaning breath retention on inhalation and /or on exhalation, is not advisable for patients at this stage until a feeling of safety has been established or that the patient is curious enough to follow new instructions. The therapist should perform the specific *pranayama* technique themself so that the patient can decide if it feels right at this time. If the patient chooses to go against it, the therapist should explore why this avoidance occurred.

There might be factors that the therapist has not initially recognised. Sometimes it is a memory and sometimes it is a physical restriction that one has not known before. For instance, septum differences in the nose are widespread and can stop the patient from performing the techniques successfully and relaxed.

Shitali Pranayama

Shitali is a very gentle form of *pranayama* and after demanding *pranayama* techniques like *Kaphalabhati*, often happily welcomed by the patient. The patient should form the lips into a small hole as if breathing through a straw. By its nature, there will be a subtle, cooling feeling experienced in the mouth, accompanied by a sweet taste.

Inhalation only or Inhalation and Exhalation with Shitali?

- If *Shitali Pranayama* is performed only by inhalation and the exhalation is without any restriction, it usually creates a pleasant feeling of refreshment.
- If *Shitali mudra* is performed during inhalation and exhalation, it is more demanding as the inhalation has to be done with a slight increasing force from the breathing muscles, the diaphragm and the abdominal area.

Shitali is very playful compared to other *pranayama* techniques, yet, it can be straining as well, depending on the time of the day practiced or the ability of the patient to use the chest muscles accordingly. It requires training and the elasticity of the chest muscles. It is suggested to stretch before the practice so that the chest feels softer in all directions. Deep tissue massage or osteopathic treatment might also be applied on the breathing muscles accordingly.

Bhastrika

Bhastrika is a powerful *pranayama* technique and should be slowly introduced to the patient. The patient should have previous experiences with *pranayama* before starting with *Bhastrika*. The inhalation mode defines speed, rhythm and performance in many *pranayama* techniques. *Bhastrika* instead focuses entirely on the exhalation rhythm. The exhalation sound is loud and like a bellow in a smith's workshop.

Variations of the breathing experiences are important, as *vata* in the nervous patient can move quickly and keeping attention is hard for the wandering mind. As the therapist has all the best intentions to create successful settings, variations are the key to a soothing session.

Variations of Bhastrika

The fingers placed at the centre of the forehead like in N*adi Shodana*

1. The practitioner closes one nostril at a time and sucks the air quickly in, expelling the air only through one nostril, then performing *ujjayi* breathing and switching sides.
2. Closing one nostril at a time for exhalation and then inhalation and switching sides of the nostril.
3. Performing four to eight strong exhalations, switching to *ujjayi* sound and starting again. To increase the challenge, *Bhastrika* can be performed together with *moola bandha.*

The therapist should instruct the repetition of the full *Bhastrika/Ujjayi* circle two to three times, guiding the patient then into a restoring *Shavasana*, which should last at least three times longer than the *Bhastrika Pranayama* breathing in total.

Shavasana and Modifications of Supported Reclining Poses

Shavasana is a powerful *Asana*, often underestimated as such and should not be mistaken as a simple relaxing pose. Variations of *Shavasana* could be necessary if the patient does not feel comfortable resting on the floor. It is not advisable to use a massage table for the breathwork as patients could faint or feel insecure on heights fall off the table. A chair, couch or something comfortable should be used if the patient cannot sit or lie on the floor with ease and comfort.

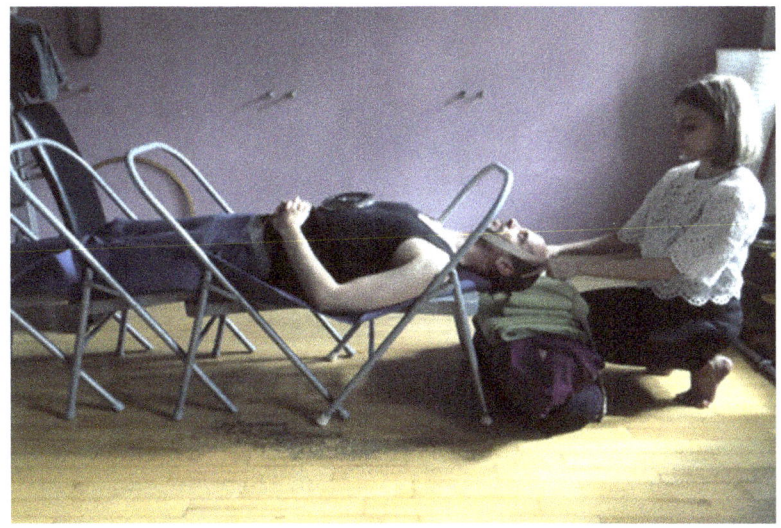

Photo: the author, assistant Romi Deift is helping a student Benjamin Martin to find a comfortable rest in *Shavasana*, supported by chairs. His neck gently extends through the pull from the yoga belts, Society of Friends, Berlin, 2019

Kaphalabhati Pranayama: *Kriya or Pranayama?*

Some people discuss if *Kapalabhati* is a type of *Pranayama* or a *Kriya*, which means it is a different practice category. However, for my research the method is now placed in the *pranayama* category, as the effects of the emotional response have been the goal of observation, not the impact on the *Srotas* or *Malas*. Like *Bhastrika Pranayama*, *Kapalabhati* deals with intense belly breathing but is less straining. The inhalation is slow and the following exhalation is forceful.

Patients and Patience

We should never push the patient into forceful breathing if any resistance or discomfort occurs or is mentioned. The patient and their experience need to be taken by the word, need to be heard and not. However, encouragement is needed as the procedure needs endurance and stamina, which is often lacking in traumatised patients. Many patients have later explained that experiencing a rise of strength or power in their bodies felt like a panic attack. The empowerment of the traumatised patient is a tricky road with unexpected turns.

When patients feel empowered and stronger, they often fear that they might be doing something wrong and are then unconsciously waiting for punishment or adverse effects. Relaxing and well-being, feeling wonderful, beautiful and loved are often desired but cannot be lived or experienced. Shame and guilt feelings often stop the patient from experiencing relaxation and pleasure. Pleasure avoidance and constant work are signs of a traumatised person.

According to my research at Society of Friends, Berlin, this was more often the case in patients who were victims emotionally or sexually in their early childhood. They were threatened with: whenever they would tell anybody, they would have to face horrible consequences. Stepping out of the acquired constant victim's position can feel very uncomfortable and challenging at first as the imprint is deep and hard to overcome.

Experiencing air hunger during breathing exercises and the urge to breathe can trigger unwanted memories. However, experiencing one could end the air hunger by simply taking a breath is a massive learning step forward to get panic under control. In the beginning, too many rounds are to be avoided as dizziness or light-headedness might occur. It is essential to plan sufficient resting times between the breathing exercise rounds and at the end of the practice.

A previously designed and well-thought-of plan often needs to be changed and played by ear according to the patient's condition and their progress during treatment. A bad night's sleep or acute emotional disturbances might need to correct the setting entirely and so does any discomfort, anger or anxiety occurring while in the breathing treatment.

Some patients also disappear from the screen for a while because they fall in love, the get ill, the move town or the feeling arises: I don't need help. It is crucial to explain the necessity for regular treatment plans and consequent self-practice. As this stage is entirely *Vata*-dominated, exhaustion of the patient might ruin the effort in making a plan in advance.

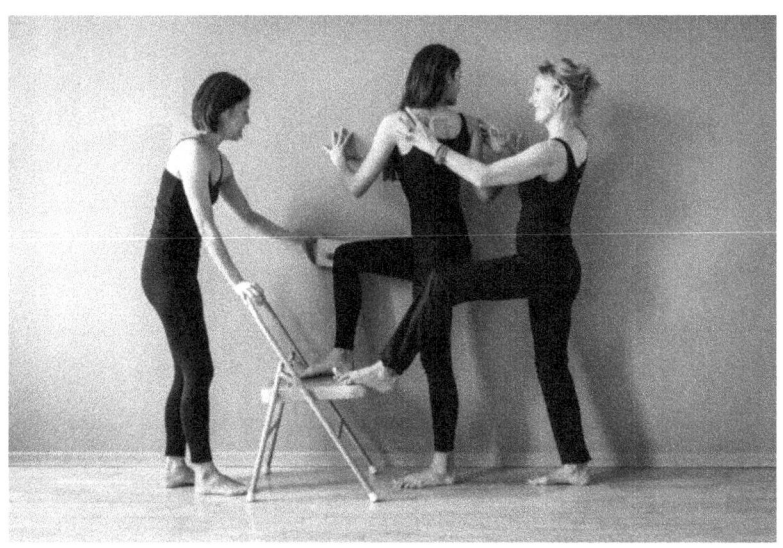

Photo: the author. Masami Kurihara and Mimi Heider de Jahnsen exploring the chest-hip relation for grounding and evolving while rotating the chest. Being rooted, supported and encouraged helps the patient stay focused on the challenge. The breath can become very restricted in this pose and eventually lead to panic attacks. These can be controlled through encouragement and empowerment of patient through the helpers. Once the patient experienced the stress relief through focused breathing, the pattern can be used in any other panic situation. Society of Friends, Berlin 2017

The Second Stage—High Tension Phase: *Pitta* dominated, fuelled by *Vata*

In the second stage of traumatic response, the patients might find themself in a constant battle of stress, threat, competition and superiority. A narcissistic personality disorder is the most common diagnosis for these patients. Not all patients, however, move to this stage. According to previously experienced traumatic experiences as well as depending on their unique *Prakriti* some patients might move on and heal after their initial exposure and through support. Some patients might skip this stage and experience straight stage 3 or 4 sensations as their inborn nature *(Prakriti)* is not allowing them to fight.

In stage 2, the quest for dominance in life's challenges is the key tool for them to survive. A constant urge to control every situation uses an enormous amount of energy. The whole mental and physical system is under stress. The patient can stay for years in this adaptation to the trauma without being diagnosed as a traumatically injured person.

Society often encourages a lifestyle that resembles the adaption of the second stage of traumatic injury: high work performance (workaholics), substance abuse or other addictive behaviour like alcoholism, shopping and sex. The addiction defines as *"behaviour that leads from short-term relief to long term negative consequences"* (Gabor Mate): "The Power of Addiction, The Addiction to Power," TED Talk, 2012 Rio, source: see Literature list.

A majority of patients at stage two of traumatic injury at my practice Society of Friends, Berlin, have been using recreational drugs on a regular base. Cocaine, speed, MDMA are the most self-prescribed recreational drugs. Ritalin is the prescribed drug that the physician had given the traumatised child diagnosed with ADD, which is the same group of substances and can cause later addiction to cocaine.

Pitta-Vata is a highly explosive mixture, fire and wind are difficult to keep under control. A feeling of a loss of control (job, relation, finances etc) can trigger sudden suicidal attempts, aggression, self-harming behaviour in action and speech or other sudden harmful decisions. The therapist should make sure that a tightly woven network of help and psychiatric aid is available at all times.

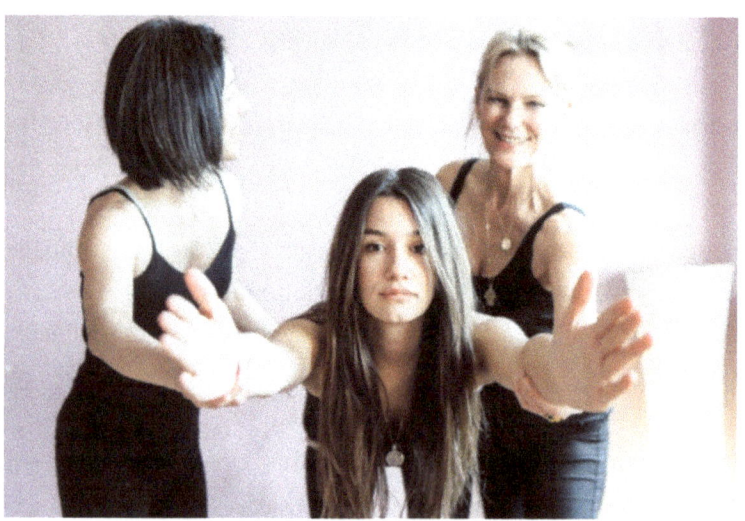

Photo: the author: students Masami Kurihara and Mimi Heider de Jahnsen are exploring *Virabdhrasana* (warrior 3) standing pose for *Pitta-Vata*. Experiencing support in a difficult pose allows the opening to trust, confidence and better compliance during treatment. Society of Friends, 2017

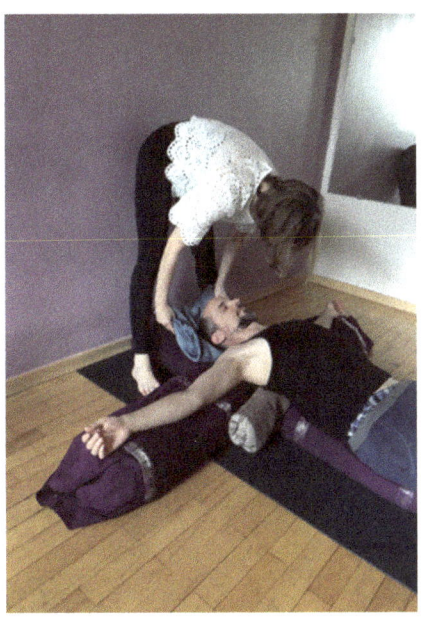

Photo: the author. Assistant Romi Deift introducing student Benjamin Martin into supported *Shavasana* variation, Society of Friends, Berlin, 2018

Shitali-Pranayama

As *Shitali Pranayama* is very sweet in taste and cooling in nature (leaving a sweet taste on the tongue), it is used when the *pitta* condition of the patient is higher than their *Vata* aspects and when it seems impossible to create any relaxing breathing pattern at all. *Shitali* captures the agitated mind through its distinct sensation in the mouth and the subtle awareness it creates. The breath should flow as if breathing through a straw by having the tongue rolled up to a thin vessel.

Variation A:

As some individuals cannot roll up the tongue, the air is sucked in through the slightly closed lips as if one is sipping hot liquid, creating a fine sharp "zsssssh." The following exhalation is soft and uncontrolled, yet the patient is encouraged to exhale as slowly and thoroughly. Slight pressure on the diaphragm should occur with an engagement of *moola bandha* or the perineum.

Variation B:

Same as above, but now the exhalation is pressed through the slightly closed lips.

So 'ham Pranayama

So 'ham is gentle until a loud, quiet or ecstatic form of sound *pranayama* meditation mantra. *So 'ham* can mean: "*so am I, I am who I am,* or even *I am Shiva.*"

Sound or Soundless: *Japa* or *Ajapa* Recitation

The sound *So* is performed on inhalation, which requires a little training.

The sound *ham* is performed on exhalation.

The practice can be either with sound (*Japa* recitation) or without sound (*Ajapa* recitation). The *Ajapa* (soundless recitation) is subtle yet beneficial at any time and can be practiced anywhere, anytime, without anyone noticing. It is helpful for patients suffering from traumatic stress syndrome to take an occasional unnoticed break—even within a meeting or on the train.

It is a secret exit door to reduce stress, decrease the heartbeat rate and reduce muscular tension in the shoulder region and lower back, mainly when practiced regularly and practiced in stressful situations. The *so ham* sound can be inhaled/exhaled in a steady rhythm for a while. The sound can increase in volume if the patient is practicing in a safe space to increase effectiveness.

Japa Recitation: Let's Get Loud

The volume of the voice can be reduced, increased, changed in whatever rhythm the patient feels comfortable and a little challenged. Variation two is to increase and decrease the speed. Variation three includes increase and decrease of speed and increase and decrease of sound.

The Third Stage: Dissociation and Denial: *Kapha, Tamas*

The therapist has to be patient with the person suffering from traumatic stress in this stage, as dissociation and denial are dominant. A strict and consequent guidance is necessary to achieve changes. Many patients in the third stage of trauma have given up. They do not feel that there is anything that could help them recover. They are even often unaware that painful experiences and shock had dulled their lives in many cases. They learned to dissociate their memories of terror from their memories in order to survive. Dissociation is always a survival mode and needs to be respected in order to heal.

One patient suffering from Fibromyalgia and chronic pain syndrome reported that she only became aware of their horrendous childhood experience after seeing a private announcement in a newspaper. She had "forgotten" what had happened.

She could not recall any events until her former class mate opened the box of Pandora. Her classmate from a Catholic boarding school in the former German Democratic Republic was looking for equally sexually assaulted children from the times she had suffered the abuse. My patient said all of a sudden she felt something like lightning going through their whole system, explaining all the constant pain she lived in all her life without knowing the cause.

In the mindset of denial, some traumatised patients are unaware that they actually live in a constant feeling of separation from their body. They live in a body and are unaware of its urges and often are emotionally stuck in a life of pleasure avoidance. They often never experienced a feeling of wholeness and integrity or they lost it during their traumatising experience. A feeling of dullness, cloudiness of the mind, forgetfulness or loss of interest in life and its fun activities has led to agony and depression as the dominating emotion.

The patients feel as if they live in a tunnel where there is no longer an expectation of a light at the end of it. The patients mostly develop a sense of rationalisation, such as "other people have difficult times too", "other people are in worse conditions", "I am not disabled, other people are"—and so forth. It is often hard introducing them to positive changes and pleasurable experiences as they often feel ashamed of their situation that objectively sometimes might not be as bad as it is experienced or they feel they do not have the right to have positive and pleasurable moments as they lost loved ones or feel too privileged.

Some patients do not allow themselves to have anything nice and comfortable done for them and strongly object to massage and any forms of kindness (see case study). The husband of one of my patients with severe major depression once said to me: " we just got back from our horse farm on our yacht and we had a fabulous holiday on our island but there is nothing that makes her happy, you instead seem to be happy without all this".

Those statements tend to put more guilt on the patients as if they are not thankful for all the beautiful things that happen to them, but if the inner mode of pleasure avoidance and pleasure denial are active through traumatic experience there is nothing that can pass through the wall of loneliness. Rationalisation provides safety. Changes that are expected, wanted, desired, encouraged are changes that lead into a world that is unknown and so changes, even if so much wanted, need a lot of courage and strong and clear support. Even if the remaining comfort zone is small, it is delivering a minimum of protection for the patient.

This needs to be understood particularly if patients in this stage do not respond accordingly to all the effort that the therapist has undertaken for a change. Keeping the patients on track is very difficult if the mind is clouded by *tamas*.

Breathing Techniques

The breathing should be carefully embedded in simple *asana* work. *Tadasana*, mountain pose, is a great pose to start with, as it can reveal its complexity and challenges by guiding the breath through the body and rediscovering body parts. By simply placing the hands on different body parts the patients can feel how the breathing movement can be directed and intensified, felt in different parts and enables them to discover and reöease tension.

If possible, the therapists can create awareness with hands-on. Some patients might respond well to touch others are very sensitive to it and feel discomfort by being touched. If it is not possible for the therapist to guide the breath with their hands, the patient is asked to apply their own hands to different body parts.

Some parts, like the region between the shoulder blades can only be reached by the therapist or a helper, but other tools like blankets or blocks, bolster can be used to apply a gently pressure. The therapist then asks the patient to direct the breath and fill the area with awareness and air.

Mental Ama Reflects Life's Burden

Taking up space in a room by filling the lungs with air, lifting arms or even moving the arms freely can be already an overwhelming experience for some patients. I guided the patients through moving smaller circles in the beginning to have pleasant experiences and gradually increased the diameters. After each intervention, resting time should be planned. The therapist should not expect positive feedback immediately. The reactions of the patients vary according to their Vkrit.

From Inside Out, Outside In

The general awareness is directed from the outside to the inside of the body, from the gross to the subtle. Everything that the patients have experienced in their life has been become a burden. It potentially translates as "mental-*Ama*."

To alter the mental state just with breathing might not be very successful, as Ama blocks the prana vaha srotas. A treatment based on Amapacana should be considered. As Professor Ram Manohar from Amrita College, Kerala, pointed out: "The best way to deal with mental *Ama* is starting with *Pancakarma*." (Private conversation at Birstein Symposium, 2019; Germany). Mental—*Ama* inhibits the patient from living new experiences.

Everything newly experienced or learned might quickly be forgotten if *tamas* or *ama* are present. Sometimes the patient might not even have given it a fair chance. Ignorance is a big stepping stone in the case of *Tamas*. It is not easy to design any template for the Third Stage as *Tamas* is blocking the free flow of *Prana*.

Everything that the therapist might have designed carefully cannot be put into practice as the patients remaining ignorant about the possibilities change could offer to them. They might not even show up or cancel. Everything is meaningless. They might not cooperate. They might not take the herbs or even practice any suggested breathing exercise. The therapist needs to be prepared that their own frustration might flare up and project this onto the patient. Sometimes it does not take much to hurt a therapist's ego. The therapist must be aware of the situation and cannot be tempted to get angry, insult or reject the patient.

Understanding that the comfort zone of a traumatised patient in *kapha* or *tamas* has been experienced as life-saving for them is crucial. The patient might feel emotionally quite stable. Suicidal attempts are rare in the Third Stage of trauma as the patients lack the energy to end their life.

Therefore, it is advisable to be very cautious with invigorating techniques. herbs that an activating like Ashvagandha or Bala can therefore increase a risk of self-harm and should only be given under strict supervision. The patient is usually under psychiatric medication (which are generally "downers") and inactive due to a depletion of *ojas*. This does not imply that nothing can be done. On the contrary, *pranayama* is a safe way to carefully and controlled enter the world of the patient's inner retreat.

Breathing into the palms and the sole of the feet

Beginning with lifting the arms into *urdhva hastasana*, repeating the position of the hands upwards, palms should be stretched and open. A subtle awareness should be created inside the hands and on the feet while the skin is stretched.

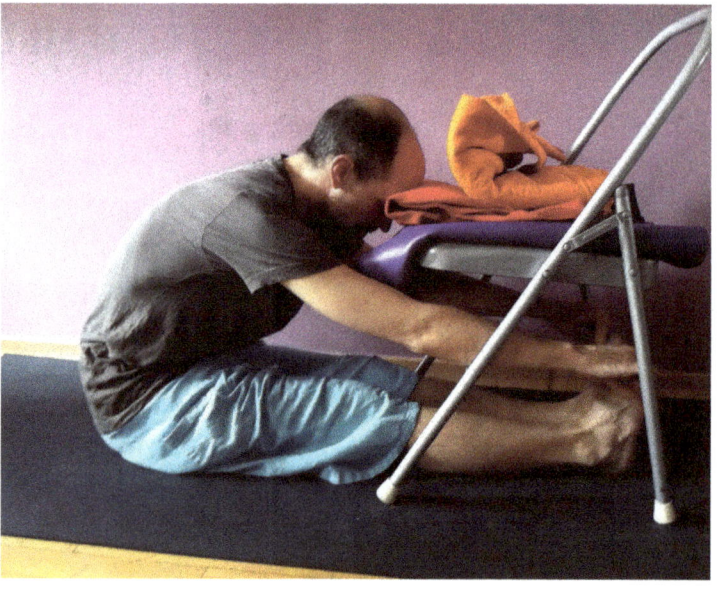

Photo: the author. Student Benjamin Martin performing relaxation pose variation for better chest breathing in a supported *pachimottasana*

Wide swinging rotations of the arms are a good way to direct the attention from the collapsed centre to the outside. When it comes to simple *pranayama* techniques, inhalation should be the main focus of attention. Inhalation is energising. Focusing on exhalation is gently and profoundly relaxing, therefore working on the vagus nerve, which leads to inactivity rather than strengthening the response to outside stimuli.

Kumbhaka, breath retention is advisable after the exhalation phase to forcefully increase the urge to inhale. Introducing the patient to air hunger is a great way to increase the intensity of the breathing and make the patient aware of how shallowly they have been breathing before.

Open your heart

So-called "heart-opening poses," better-called backbends, like *Ushtrasana* (camel pose), work on the feeling of courage and stability. They can be supported with blankets and bolsters to challenge the patient comfortably. Simply having the chest supported with a blanket, bolster or block stabilises, lifts mood and can be practiced alone at home. A small yoga wheel, an Iyengar yoga backbend tool or a bolster can intensify the gentle opening without pain or strain.

Brhmari Pranayama:

Brhmari is best performed in a small group as the soothing humming sound intensifies and works more effectively in an acoustically supportive group. Tamboora, Sitar or Harmonium background sounds can be used if this is not possible. The patient sits comfortably on the floor or a chair, bolster or couch and inhales gently. They start making a humming sound on exhalation while closing their eyes, ears and lips with their fingers. If this creates a feeling of disorientation, the patient can comfortably keep the hands resting on the lap and start to close either ears or eyes after sometime of practice.

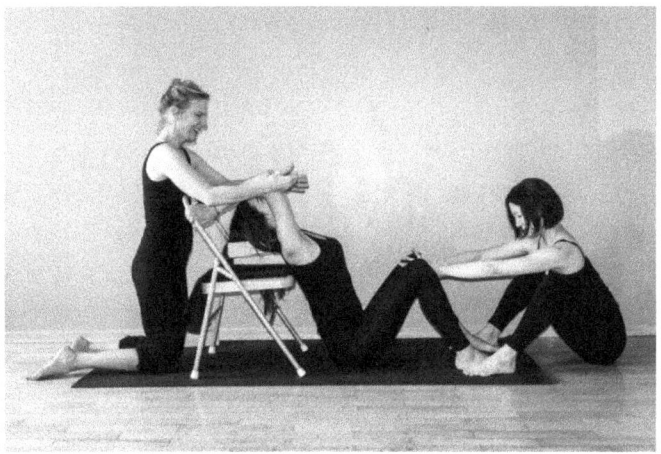

Photo: the author. Students Masami Kurihara and Mimi Heider de Jahnsen are exploring the breath-relaxation axis in a supported back band, called "a heart-opener." Society of Friends, Berlin, 2017

Summary and Research Presentation of Society of Friends, Berlin In The Years 1996-2020

As I had the chance to carefully study and analyse the therapeutic work approaches on Post Traumatic Stress Disorder / Trauma of the last 40 years, the power of breath work has been underestimated. By doing so, a profound, effective and affordable treatment method has been missed. Particularly communities with low income can benefit from a method that can be used even independently from the medical system and its generally high priced methods.

If I could think of a dream, it is the one of educating people in local communities as breath workers and thereby creating networking breathing therapists for low income or remote living groups. During the work on my project for the European Union on "Accompanying the Dying, Intercultural Studies and help" and "Massage, Meditation and Mindfulness".

It showed clearly that migrant groups, minorities and people with PTSD backgrounds, often overlapping, brought so much competence with them that it was easy to use these resources to educate them as therapists. The intimate knowledge of culture and of coping mechanisms within cultures was more helpful and direct to the point than what psychotherapists in Germany could offer.

When it comes to finding a psychotherapist in Germany, it is just by good luck to meet a therapist that is specialised in trauma. Many misleading encounters before finding a therapist can prolong an efficient treatment for years of suffering.

In my experience, psychotherapists have not often volunteered for education in breathing techniques as a profound part of therapy. Some might have felt that it is not "a real thing" because, of course, every one of us breathes naturally. Yet this is not the whole story. To understand the methods and effects of *pranayama* breath work, therapists should give it a go in self-experience, understand the need to self-practice.

Whenever we trained breath work assistants at Society of Friends, Berlin, they observed the subtle changes in their minds and well-being through *pranayama* already within the first days of practice. They reported that it was not as easy as they had expected, that it was challenging, but the immediate effects were so convincing that they continued the daily routine for their own good. They also reported the positive changes they observed in themselves by simply guiding the patients through the practice.

Pranayama can be easily learned and practiced. It is a gentle and safe form of intervention—safe to apply (with the mentioned precautions) and results are far easier to achieve than in a meditation practice. Meditation needs long-term continuous training and preparation for months and even years to effect.

As Prof. Ram Manohar mentioned that for people with mental issues like depression, PTSD and other, meditation can be counter—productive. Meditation, he states, is for only for the healthy individual.

From my personal experience with patients who suffered from PTSD and tried meditation, I strongly support Prof. Ram Manohar's caution. I want to add the experience that unfortunately several patients who participated in intense meditation retreats (like *Vipassana* in the name of S.N. Goenka, Burmese—Indian teacher, 1924-2013) reported mental states of dissociation and sleeplessness after the retreat.

These disturbances led in one known case even to suicidal attempts. I therefore promote a safe and simple method of controlled breathing which is less demanding, straining and can be monitored by an experienced practitioner for a long time ahead.

Footnote:

As I am a free diver (apnea diving) and study pranayama, I was surprised how free divers use much scientific knowledge to improve their performance. One can stay underwater longer if deep relaxation is achieved and every possible relaxation method is used. In pranayama, we discovered a technique that can relax a person deeply and almost instantly.

I work with young patients suffering from PTSD and cooperate with free dive instructors. I successfully sent the patients into beginners' free-diving classes of Static Apnea. Static apnea is an easy way to explore breath, pranayama, the source of fear, how to relax—method: The diver is floating freely on water, wearing floats and neoprene, goggles and nose clip and is holding the breath on inhalation or exhalation.

There is no movement involved in static apnea, unlike other free-diving disciplines like free immersion, no fins, distance etc. The body uses larger amounts of oxygen when there is tension anywhere in the muscles. Through body scanning during the floating, the diver learns to detect tense spots and to release them consciously in order hold the breath longer. The diver can only achieve a better result by deeper relaxation.

In particular, for young people breath training, performance and deep relaxation training, all coming in one attractive package as a competitive sport instead of sessions with a psychiatrist, which, of course, should never be substituted or replaced without proper evaluation of the case. My patients were excited as they felt hope and not left out. Floating in prone position in a wet suit in blood temperature water, counting seconds and controlling bodily tension as well as the urge to breathe they reported, was transforming.

This free-diving technique I used so far particularly for Pitta patients who could not calm down successfully and were little responsive to the idea of yoga. Some went for deep line diving (diving down into depths around 8-25 meters with no oxygen supply, just by holding the breath) and reported that they now manage to control suicidal attempts much better. In my experience, understanding the breath and learning how to use it beneficially in order to heal is understanding the body-mind relation on a clear experimental level that leads to positive experiences.

Small Steps: The "Breath-Self-Study—Plan"

Most of my patients have shown high compliance for months which clearly documents their interest in the method and that the method itself was a convincing and promising treatment to step out of panic, anxiety, guilt and shame. They reported that they felt better, calmer and made better choices, were less forgetful.

Layout of the Research Study Based on *Pranayama* at Society of Friends, Berlin

—first thing in the morning: the patients are supposed to start with the *pranayama* as part of the *Dinacharya,* their daily routine, slowly and gently inhaling and exhaling, feeling the breath moving inside the body like wind on a landscape.

—After a minimum of three breathing cycles, they hold the breath on inhalation and document the time, then repeat the same, this time after a full exhalation.

The training's effects are usually seen within two days of practice. After one week, the self-study effect becomes clear: the patients experience that on certain days the breathing is more restricted, the chest feels tight, while on other days, immediately after waking up, everything is easy and they enjoy the smooth start into the day.

- The patients send a daily text message with the timing, which will be commented on. Comments are supposed to be encouraging.
- If the result are under the estimated results, we will be suggest to take it easy. If the result shows improvements, we encourage the patients to enjoy their strength.
- All patients and students who participated in the program reported that they found repetitive patterns in their emotional response during their daily emotional responses in relation to their morning breathing performance. They started their inquiries out of curiosity.
- The diary of practice showed that repetitive pattern can be observed, like: chickpeas and ice cream for a late night dinner, bad sleep, next day emotionally upset, craving coffee and sweets, feeling guilty and unstable. More diligently practice showed them that they achieved a calmer and better start position into the day with more training and understanding patterns of avoidance as much as patterns of indulgence.
- They reported that they became more receptive to the change of breath and their ability to alter stressful situations by breath awareness and breath control.
- Some tried holding their breath after a stressful situation or after a happy day and so on so forth. From there, the patients developed a more profound interest in the power of *pranayama* and started a deeper practice.

More Tests: The Blood Pressure/ Breathing Relation

The Society of Friends, Berlin treatment team researched experienced yoga teachers exposed to stressful situations while measuring the pulse and blood pressure. As stressful situation for the trial had to be found that is easy to induce and not harmful. So we decided to use the headstand (shirsasana) model. Shirasana in a supported version, can be practiced by anyone without the need of detailed previous instructions. As we worked with experienced yoga teachers, we did not expect any problems in this position as it is widely practiced and in most styles a preposition to becoming yoga teacher.

Observation of their breath before, during and after the stress.

1. We took the average result from their BP results in a relaxed state. The same procedure was used for the pulse rate. The used BP monitor shows the pulse rate accurately. The breathing was observed at all times. All measurements were done three times with a simple electronic BP monitor by the company Omron.

2. The student was asked to go into a relaxed, supported, *Shirshasana* position (headstand pose).

BP and pulse were measured three times and then the middle result was taken as a test result.

The relaxed *Shirshasana* / headstand pose was possible through a defined assist in the pose. The student brought their head in between the folded hands on the floor. The shoulders rested on the legs of a helper who was seated behind the student. A second assistant lifted the test person's legs until they were parallel to the floor and the helper kept them lifted during the procedure. This assist made sure that not too much weight is distributed on the upper arms, which would have caused an increase in blood pressure. So, we could identify the experienced stress or distress without the muscular strain on the forearm.

3. The students then return to the previous *Shavasana* position, resting on the floor and relaxing. Again, blood pressure and pulse were controlled.

The original test was published by Roqcue Lobo in the 70 is, where he challenged yoga teachers, athletes and untrained people in upside down positions and published his research.

During his study, Lobo had included Echocardiograms, oxygenation level and other vital parameters, like measuring directly at the heart, which we could not reproduce in our clinical trial. The outcome:

- athletes had shown an increase in BP as well as
- untrained people (40 mmHg or above), while

- Yoga practitioners and yogis had shown a steady BP or a minor increase (below or equal 20mmHg).

    Lobo concluded that athletes and untrained people showed signs of distress during the headstand and need more time to recover than yoga practitioners who experienced a deeper relaxation.

For my study at my practice, Society of Friends, Berlin the measurements of vital parameters were reduced to a few of Lobo's and other, more practical measurements were introduced. The focus was set on measuring BP, pulse rate, oxygenation and breath observation. The key tool to induce deep relaxation was to slow down the breath rate and to control the diaphragm by consciously relaxing all breathing muscles, all working muscles, particularly the trapezius.

The trapezius muscle is one of the most critical distress indicators. Located in the back shoulders, spreading out to the skull, the outer shoulder, the shoulder blades and then covering the thoracic and the cervical spine. The trapezius contracts in any stressful situation. The modern lifestyle that makes us spend most hours sitting and looking at screens or holding onto steering wheels.

Our lifestyle is demanding in a fight-or-flight response that mostly is unnecessary, like in a traffic jam. Our posture freezes in stress, keeping unproportioned tension in the shoulder girdle. Chronic pain syndromes and destruction of the cervical spine already at a young age are the result of lifestyle that is merely sympathicoton (Pitta—Vata) and rajasic opposed to a healthy Vagus dominant life style (sattvic Pitta).

The reduction of pain during our study was often the first success felt by my patients. Even if in the beginning a tenderness in the affected areas was felt. We explained that a chronic tension in the muscle is actually a constant activity— the pain after release is the same pain one experiences after a heavy workout. It is lactic acid and inflammation bodies released into the blood stream. The pain could be reduced by ice packs or sometimes Paracetamol (500mg).

The Outcome of the Study on *Pranayama*, Stress and Relaxation via BP/Pulse by Society of Friends, Berlin on yoga teachers:

- 90% of the students showed an increase of the BP that was far too high.
- their BP increased over 40mm Hg and the pulse rate increased over 40 beats/min.

- only one experienced teacher showed an average increase of only 23 mm Hg.
- one student with regular meditative and yoga practice showed an increase of only 30mm Hg after two years of intense studies.

Conclusion

Many modern western yoga styles, particularly *Vinyasa Yoga* (a form of yoga where the speed of changes from one *asana* to the next is merely on a single breath), do not reach the goal of introducing changes to the body-mind connection. Fitness work outs might contribute to longevity and better health, but not necessarily to stress control.

However, meditation and *asana* work clearly do. Most yoga teachers have been performing *asanas* as poses of bodywork instead of understanding the essence of the figure. Learning that asanas are stressful positions for the body that teach the student transforming stress into deep relaxation. They remained in a state of ambition and competition and showed physical signs of an increased stress response. A *rajas* mind can enter the stage of *sattva* by control of the *vrittis*.

- After the stressful situation, the tested yoga teachers and students still showed signs of distress. They needed long to relax their bodies, which could easily be shown by their vital parameters in their blood pressure, breathing and pulse rate.
  Continuing studies at Society of Friends, Berlin had shown that through sensitive and diligent practice of *pranayama* and other breathwork can result in long-lasting changes in the stress response and control.
- Therefore, *pranayama* and all other breathwork methods can contribute to stress control and mental health and can be part of any other treatment.
- *Pranayama* can help to overcome or control PTSD symptoms like dissociation, depression, anxiety and sleep disorders.
- The correct choice of *pranayama* techniques is important for safe treatment. There is no universal *pranayama* prescription.
- A fundamental knowledge of ayurveda and yoga and serious self-practice is needed for a successful treatment.
- Therapists should have self—experience to understand the changes and possibilities and the effects themself.

Panc Karma at Society of Friends: Treatment Options for Mental and Physical Recovery After Traumatic Injuries and in PTSD

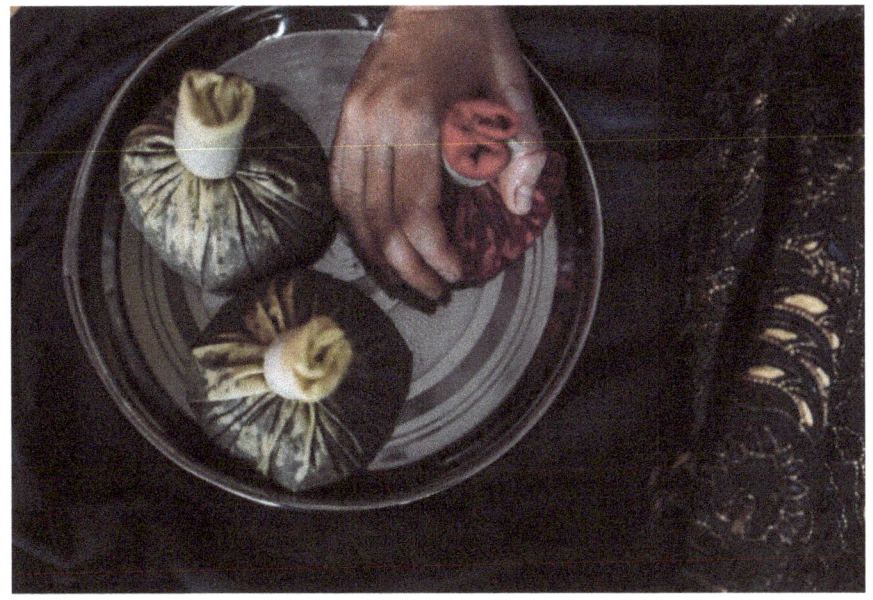

Photo: Dr Anastasia Shchedrina performing Pizzhili on a patient,
Photo credit: Natalia Smirnova, 2019

Over the years, *Panc Karma* has become the primary treatment system at Society of Friends. At least one-third of the patients participate in at least one *Panc Karma* annually, as they enjoy the benefits that occur each time.

We hosted monthly *Panc Karma* treatments .

An average of eight to nine guests were invited to stay for the phase of *Snehana* (inner Olation), leading to some over 800 patients in the last years.

Most of the treated patients had been patients of Society of Friends, Berlin, before the decision to experience a more profound, more intensive treatment. Due to the restrictions for therapists and practices during the pandemic, we decided to offer one-to-one settings.

A great influence in the new setting is Mrs Dr Anastasia Shchedrina, who works in Malaga, Spain, and Tel Aviv, Israel, with our patients in the new format while I myself work in Berlin, Germany, and on call. Our *Pancakarma* settings can be applied anywhere in almost a pop-up standard, providing all the important tools and techniques to lead a successful *Panc Karma.*

The pre-*Panc Karma* treatment consisted of *Amapachana* and *Agni* invigoration with various herbs:

Mustha, Citrak or Pippali carefully selected according to the patient's condition and lifestyle.

Vamana treatment plus medication and *abhyanga* application turned out to significantly reduce anxiety, suicidal attempts, insomnia, agitation and guilt.

Exclusion measures at Society of Friends, Berlin:

- Unknown patients that approached via website
- Patients that were disrespectful during their past treatments
- Patients with significant personality disorders and a history of violence
- Patients who continued recreational drugs during *amapachana* treatment
- Patients who refused to have a biomedical check-up before the treatment
- Patients who had a suicidal attempt in the weeks before the treatment
- Patients who suffered from loneliness, as well as those with social phobia
- Patients who started anti-depressive medication less than three months before the *Panc Karma*. As the Ghee might interact with the absorption of the anti-depressant drugs, it is advisable to exclude patients under medication or contact the psychiatrist to interrupt the intake.

Observations on Traumatised Patients Undergoing *Pancakarma* and *Purva Karma* at Society of Friends.

At my practice Society of Friends, Berlin some patients suffering from PTSD were chosen to participate in a full *Panckarma* treatment. The patients started with a two-week program of *Agni sara*. The patients had to obey a strict food and lifestyle regimen during these two weeks. These restrictions led to various unexpected problems. 60-80 per cent of the patients emphasised that they had experienced unusual anger.

Those anger episodes happened particularly when they felt disturbed in their thoughts or asked to be social. Some patients reported problems in sticking to a plan at all. They said, experiencing any restrictions or guidelines were triggering for them. However, this can be true, but it can also be a sign of not wanting to change.

Therefore, we prefer patients that we already worked with in the past so there is a bond of trust established. None of these problems occurred with patients that we had previously known for years of treatment. Prof. Gupta, Nadiad, India, only works with the Pippali *Amapacana* concept with indoor patients, which makes totally sense in my eyes, as particularly western patients do have a tendency to not follow the rules strictly enough.

Again, the traumatised patients might have to struggle with restrictions and often faces difficulties to welcome a change. It is important to understand that it is not the patient to be blamed, but the setting that has to be changed to overcome those mental obstacles. Some of the patients reported that they were more focused on themselves in the sense of calmness and self-care. Part of frustration as well as part of the improvement, was the time-consuming food preparation.

After some days, though, they experienced relief and reported staying more focused, exploring their own needs and the connection to what they eat became important.

Some patients with eating disorders wanted to stop the diet, as they felt they had become more irritable and bad-tempered in the beginning due to the regular meal system. These symptoms subsided after a while when those patients adapted to the lifestyle changes.

Changing a lifestyle is demanding and challenging and needs a lot of trust in the time ahead and the company on the way, which is the therapist. Patients who were always up for a "hit" had to learn slowly and patiently to stay quiet, talk less, not to party enjoy walks in nature or read a book instead of constantly pulling all strings at once. During the following *Pancakarma* intern treatment, those patients often experienced drastic emotional changes again.

Being in a controlled environment under constant supervision, being told what to do, what not to do or not to rest, increased adverse feelings. Mostly these feelings subsided after the second or third day they allowed themselves to feel good, accept the massages and accept the food and care.

Most of them then reported a decrease of being bloated and an increased feeling of sensitivity in the guts and emotional stability after. Their sleep clearly improved in all study participants, lustrous skin, emotional regulation, regulation of appetite, increase of wellbeing, increase of positive physical feelings. A new sense of serenity, calmness, inner quietness and a feeling of satisfaction and a new feeling of a meaning in life was mentioned repeatedly.

One of the patients asked if they could continue the regimen for at least another six weeks, as they felt relieved not to be involved in daily activities as before. They felt relieved not being responsible for the changes in their lifestyle as they had the prescription or the order from my practice. Those prescriptions are: "no decision making", "don't get involved in other people's problems as you are now vulnerable and need the time for self-recovery (emotional dieting)", "no sex", "no heavy carrying"" as little movement as possible".

Those are indisputable rules to follow. All decisions or any problem-solving are supposed to be postponed for the following weeks (if the issues still existed). Patients felt relieved and discovered that a lot of their daily stress was not necessary as they often acted as people pleaser instead of living their own life, took too many duties on board, were afraid to be called lazy or inefficient.

Emotional Trauma: Observed Behavioural Pattern According to *Doshas* Under *Pancakarma* Treatment at Society of Friends, Berlin, 2000-2022

The following table shows my observation of dosha—related patterns of behaviour before and often during treatment. None of these patterns should stop the therapist from booking in a patient, however, just be aware and alert of the frequently seen typical problems that can occur. Once on knows, it is easy to be prepared and continue the treatment without unwanted side effects. Pancakarma is definitely a high profiled treatment chance that should not be missed as the benefits for the patients are long lasting and often life-changing.

Vata	Pitta	Kapha
Recent Traumatic injury or the traumatising situation has happened repeatedly childhood	Traumatic injury 10-20 years prior to symptoms	Adaption to the traumatic events by dissociation and ignorance. Often underlying childhood abusive traumatic injuries followed by abusive relationships, miscarriages
Strategy of avoidance in daily life and in PK: Tendency to collapse, emotionally	Strategies of avoidance: in daily life an under treatment: dominance, flirting, anger,	Strategy of avoidance in daily life and under treatment: dull thinking, unfocused mind, numbing, helpless, demanding

unstable and fragile, mood swings, crying, eating disorders, breaking the rules with the excuse of exhaustion	arguing, drug abuse, alcoholism, verbally abusive, bad jokes on behalf of others, manipulating, complaining and breaking rules	"oral" structural behaviour, complaining, not changing
Emotional: unsatisfied, rough and abrupt behaviour, easily and suddenly startled, crying, shouting, whispering constantly changing, new symptoms occurring, anxiety	Emotional: easy to upset. Blaming others. Intake of alcohol or drugs before, after and even under treatment, blaming others for discomfort	Emotional: dissociated, interrupted by tiredness and disinterest, laziness.
Changing attitude, lack of trust, self-prescribing herbs, distraction via social media	Argumentative, need to be in control, self—prescribed changes of the treatment. Threatening to leave and blame the staff	Hopeless, negative thoughts, feeling of being in a dark place with no way out, lying down despite being told to stay up, day sleep
Unsocial, arriving late or interrupting the treatment, breaking up or other ways to boycott by not following the rules and regulations for safety. Anal behaviour.	Doing too many things at the same time: being on the computer, phone, still working, cannot relax, high tension, narcissistic attention seeking, dominant behaviour in the group, criticising the staff and the treatment in front of others, joking about the procedures, not taking the treatment seriously	Doing very little. Demanding help for almost everything, untidy. Unclean, untidy, oral comfort, creating more work for the staff without noticing, feeling of not being involved in the process
Impatient, fragile, shaking, tremors, feeling cold, discomfort in lying down, sitting up just anything. Nothing is right	Sudden aggression, headaches, increasing pain syndromes	Falling asleep

forgetful	Knowing everything better, manipulative	Not interested in anything
Has not bought the medicine, forgot to take the medicine, took it according what was falsely remembered. lost the notes	Has bought the medicine, pricy high medicine and taking double the amount.	Has bought the medicine, too much of it, but cannot be motivated to take it. Can't find it.
Difficulty in following any rule because of lack of concentration, messy, material not available, ADHD	Difficulty in following the rules because of doubts "that this works" and needs to be in control, narcissism	Difficulty in following the rules because of lack of effort, not showing up, laziness, lack of motivation, depression

Conclusion:

The importance of *Pancakarma* treatment for PTSD and related psychological disorders like addiction became evident through the beneficial results for the patients.

The improvement of self-care was the most important marker, often represented by the change in addictive behaviour/substance abuse, improvement of sleep, overall happiness.

- 99% of the patients quit smoking, even without having had a primary intention to do so! (in more than 800 patients, only three people continued smoking during the procedures and those were the ones that continued smoking tobacco)
- 80% reported a significant decrease in the use of recreational drugs like cocaine for at least three months
- 85% reported more self-care in eating habits for at least three months
- 60% reported an improvement of sleep over five months period
- 85% reduced their intake of painkillers and asthma sprays
- 60 % felt lighter and happier for five months follow up
- 90% of bulimic patients reported a significantly reduced urge to vomit under stress. For them, a particular treatment plan with induced *vamana* (vomiting) was created that introduced a feeling of disgust to self-induced vomiting.

Every second patient has already been a patient at my practice Society of Friends, Berlin and decided with the team that a more profound step towards health and wellbeing was necessary. Trust, safety and confidence need to build up with patients who have PTSD, which can take a while. New patients mainly arrived through recommendations. Advertising the retreats was avoided to keep the patient groups relatively small and intimate.

Patients of such different needs and health issues, starting from cancer to multiple sclerosis and PTSD, the qualified staff and the special small setting had proven it right to do so. Patients with special needs, like those suffering from cancer, Multiple sclerosis, Diabetes, Bi-Polar will receive an adapted program and one should be able to work with a well-trained and educated staff.

As Charaka states that one of the pillars of healing is the medical staff, I am opposing to weekend training courses for ayurveda therapists without a profound knowledge. I think if doctors from other continents would arrive, do a weekend surgery and then offer to operate we would easily feel that this is inappropriate, for ayurveda it is the same: it is a complex medical system that can provide treatments that are sharp and precise like a scalpel.

Patients mostly repeated our *Pancakarma* within 12 months, some even every three to four months, as they experienced support and realised their wish to change habits was pretty stress free and nicely supported. In the case of drug addiction, the results are mostly shown after two or three *Pancakarma* treatments. A significant reduction mainly had been reported after the first *Pancakarma*.

The accessibility of Society of Friends located in the centre of Berlin as an urban centre and the constant availability of the staff created a safe space for continuity work. After relapse, there was always an option to find help within days.

All patients who quit smoking, using cocaine or other high addictive drugs reported no withdrawal symptoms at all. Only two patients continued smoking during the treatment and continued after. All other patients reportedly had no unpleasant effects like withdrawal symptoms after quitting.

This observation lead to assumption that suffering or withdrawal symptoms of any drug are not the master way to cure addiction although it is the psychiatric gold standard. Guilt, shame, pain, hopelessness and suffering through drug detoxification (cold turkey) do not prevent a relapse. But care, love and safety are more likely to do so. I observed hundreds of patients suffering from addiction and reporting how awful the several detoxification programs had been, how painful, how humiliating.

Many of them I still see decades later. They said that the loving kindness they had received in the practice and the confidence we had in them were the better help. They felt we were able to restore self-worth, self-acceptance by treating them respectfully, even in times of relapse. Many addicts told me years later that they actually had gone through difficult times when we met and that they were ashamed to tell me.

Realising later on that they actually started using less and changed their lifestyle in their own mode without us imposing a new lifestyle or criticising them. It was particularly the welcoming atmosphere and the total acceptance they received that later they said it was the key for their recovery.

The Method

The exceptionally kind and caring attention that the patient receives during *Pancakarma* seems to be in a contrast to the strong elimination methods during the retreat(the five—panc-karma—actions) like vomiting, enemas, blood-letting, sweat, steam, etc., sound pretty unpleasant. However, the patients all reported clear relief, reduced tension and reduced discomfort in the body and mind: "*as if a monster was leaving the body*" Patient J., 2019. The staff treated the patients as gentle as nature, kind, almost nurturing and motherly. The patients felt accepted, not judged.

As Ashkan Sepahvand said: *You never said: I was a mess like you, but then I became better, I saw I was ignorant and now I am such a better person than you. This is what other therapists do and it puts me off.* 2020, private conversation.

Description sheet for *Pancakarma* treatment for western patients in Berlin, Germany, at Society of Friends, Berlin

Your PANCAKARMA Treatment

The *Pancakarma* is an ancient traditional individual cure program.

It can be used as a program to promote well-being and relaxation, infertility treatment and treat recurring migraines or other pain syndromes like chronic back pain. It is advised after injuries and surgery and helps deal with allergies, stress and depression. It is also part of an ayurveda healing programme for chronic and severe conditions, such as Multiple Sclerosis, cancer or auto-immune diseases like Rheumatoid Arthritis.

Pancakarma is a treatment of very high value and has to be performed precisely according to the patient's condition.

You will be our guest for almost six weeks in total, yet not staying with us at all times! But we will be there to guide you through these exceptional weeks.

It is about you!

After detailed information about lifestyle and food habits provided by you over two weeks, your general health, health complaints or illness, digestive strength and moods, we decide what pre-cleansing program (*Amapachana*) will be the best preparation treatment.

1st step: AMAPACHANA

For best results of the *Pancakarma* a consultation previously to the retreat is absolutely necessary. Here, the individual amount of herbs and the duration of the first phase is set up.

Amapachana is the first stage of removing *Ama* and increasing your digestive fire.

We will be using either *Pippali, Chitrak or Mustha* powder (*churna*) according to your *Pakriti* (individual constitution) and your *Vikriti* (individual disturbance /illness/*dosha* imbalance) in an individually designed treatment plan. We will explain to you the amount of the specific *churna*. We need to receive a daily text message from you during this treatment to have a close follow-up!

During this first phase, it is recommended to see us 2-3 times for a check-up on pulse and tongue and applications such as the *Udvarthana* massage plus steam bath or infrared sauna.

Most of the preparations that we will recommend can also be done alone at home, like:

—long warm or cold showers

—daily dry scrub massage

—or other individually suggested methods.

Every day, please, send us a brief report via text message to 49-179 73 78210 about:

1. Headache: where, when and how? 1-10 pain scale
2. Body aches and pain, where and how? 1-10

3. General feeling: 1-10
4. Digestive power, appetite, hunger 1-10 changes?
5. Stool: colour, odour, consistency? Descriptive, please, no photos.
6. Sleep: Times and Hours
7. Sleep: Quality 1-10
8. Dreams
9. Energy
10. Mood
11. Other remarks, etc.

During this first phase, make sure that you are getting adequate rest.

No sports are allowed, including biking, horseback riding and yoga. Sex is not allowed, too. In short terms: all activities you have your mouth open and disturb your regular breathing pattern. If you have a specific question, be free to ask at any time.

No physical and mental excitement. Stay away from decision-making or problem-solving. Keep clear for 14 weeks of all extra stress. Yes, it is possible.

Light exercises are fine. Strolls in the park. Avoid excessive or loud talking, arguments or mental stress.

Enjoy light cooked meals, preferably home-cooked, soups and porridges, best with rich with ghee or organic oils. In case of eating out, Italian restaurants are nothing but trouble, yet most Indian or Vietnamese restaurants provide suitable food.

Strictly avoid raw vegetables, juices, dairy products (not milk!), legumes, fried or baked food.

Avoid travel and unnecessary stays outside in the cold, wind or direct sunshine.

Wear a hat and scarf. After meals, do not expose yourself to sunshine. Day sleep is not suggested, yet a bit of snoozing is fine.

Have at least 6 hours of sleep, best before midnight, suggested is 10 PM (YES!).

Keep sufficiently warm and comfortable at all times.

Enjoy the subtle changes. Enjoy yourself.

2nd step: **PURVAKARMA**—external preparation
SNEHANA—olation

SVEDANA—sweating

The hot phase!

Thursday

We will take care of you and everything that has to be done. Please, plan the following days. Schedule your life so you can enjoy the next days in a calm and relaxed state till Sunday evening.

Inform friends and family that you are in a retreat and you might be offline. Give them my number so that they feel comfortable.

It is an intense treatment, so all emotional disturbances should wait. Always keep in mind: you are doing this for yourself. If you are feeling happy and healthy, you will spread joy.

We roll:

All participants gather for the first dinner with ghee—drinking—your amount of ghee will be adapted to your *dosha* disturbance.

The Gayatri Mantra accompanies us for the period of the cure.

Om Bhur bhuva Svaha
Om tat Savitur varenyam
Bhargo devasya dhimahi
Dhiyo yo nah pracodayat.

It is an appeal to heaven to bestow upon us with wisdom and insight.

We will be rechecking all the important information:

—blood pressure

—digestion

—appetite

—signs and symptoms according to your inner *snehana*

—nausea

—headaches

—sleep

—emotions

—power

Saturday and Sunday are directed individually according to different symptoms during the cleaning process.

Those symptoms can be increased appetite, yawning, headache or nausea, spontaneous vomiting or severe tiredness or no particular symptoms at all.

The unpleasant symptoms are generally not present when you respect to rest. You are not sleeping during the day, especially right after meals. Do not take any stimulants such as coffee or nicotine. Even staying outside in the wind, rain or direct sunshine can produce adverse effects. Every physical strain should be avoided to have the most benefit and the least unwanted side effect.

Please, strictly AVOID for your own good:
Daytime sleep
Sex
Staying outdoors
Food, other than the provided or recommended
Raw vegetables/fruit/juice
Coffee, alcohol, nicotine, chocolate
Crying, shouting, anger
Too much speaking
Phone calls/emails
Arguments, troubles
Rides and journeys
Hot baths
Cold baths
Sports
Exciting literature or films, including sex books
Exposure to wind, rain, sun, cold, heat
Facial and body creams not given
Recreational drugs
*Prescribed medication should resume use.

For your own interest: during the four days of *Pancakarma Snehana* phase, do not smoke or drink alcohol or deviate from the diet recommendations.

All participants will be interviewed again in the morning and evening about how they feel, how their digestion might have changed and other symptoms.

For example, the amount of ghee you will be drinking could change or finish.

In some cases, it is suggested to continue the ghee drinking for a certain amount of time after the *Pancakarma*.

Envy is inappropriate. Sometimes you might want the same treatment as your friend, but it could be a wrong choice (!) or you think you are not getting enough ghee.

There will be various ayurveda treatments performed on Saturday and Sunday. Depending on pre-existing conditions or complaints, your individual program will be designed.

The powders and oils used for your health and comfort are produced according to the traditional rules of ayurveda. All products are bought from reliable and tested sources like Ayurveda Handel Hamburg, Herr Wolfgang Keicher.

They are free of chemicals,f reshly prepared. Allergy-risky herbs like Neem are avoided.

Following treatments might be performed during the Pancakarma:

Udvartana—powder massage

Garshana—silk glove massage

Snehana—oiling

Padabhyanga—foot Massage

Shiroabhyanga—head massage

Abhyanga—full body oiling

Mukhabhyanga—face olation treatment

Annalepa—application of mud

Karnapurnam—ear oiling

Pizhili—warm oil treatment

Tapa Sveda—hot, dry wrap

Patra Pinda Sveda Potali—hot herbal wrap

Pinda svedana—hot oil stamps

Nasatarpana—nose oiling

Shirodhara—warm forehead flowing olation

Akshitarpana—eye oiling, milk massage

Svedana—steam bath

And more—

After the completed digestion of the ghee, the five actions (literal translation of *Pancakarma*) will be performed: (yet not all of them are necessarily performed by each patient):

Vamana—vomiting (rarely indicated)

Virecana—removal through the intestine

Anuvasana and *Niruha Vasti*—enemas

Snehana Nasti—nose therapy

Raktamokshana—bloodletting (rarely indicated)

On Sunday evening, most of the participants will have completed the *snehana* (inner olation) phase and will have been able to perform some of the above listed.

Sign of the complete digestion of fat:

lustrous eyes

a feeling of lightness

complete digestion with light stool; almost no paper is needed!

no headaches

improved sense of smell

improved eyesight

soft elastic, baby-like skin

reduction of wrinkles around the eyes

a feeling of rest and peace

good appetite

good night sleep

a general feeling of wellbeing and happiness

3rd Step: **ELIMINATION**

Monday

Monday is a rest day for you (you can go to work, depending on what you do).

Eat very little, preferably a light watery rice soup.

On Monday night we apply the enema. If you do not have time, take it easy and complete it within the following days.

Get an irrigator from the pharmacy or online. The watery preparation is made of 1 litre of water and a handful of *Dashamool* herbs. Boil down the infusion to ½ L. We will provide the herbs.

Allow it to cool down to blood temperature (test this on your wrist)

For the application, lie on your right side. If the enema is completely emptied, turn your body onto the left side and wait patiently. Retain the enema as long as possible. A hot water bottle helps against cramps occurring.

In uncertain patients, instead, an enema Microklist could be used (pharmacy).

4th step: **RASAYANA—Rejuvenation**
Slowly dive back into your life.

In this phase, which can last up to one hundred days, individual applications with medicated oils, *pranayama*, yoga, showers, herbal preparations and lifestyle plans will guide you

Enjoy life, enjoy health and happiness!

We are there for you!

Bring your sincere motivation and smile! Some relaxing books or games to play and share.

☺

Leave your sorrows and electronics at home.

We are looking forward to having you here!

Manuela and Team!

Please confirm with your signature that you have carefully read the above and agreed to terms, conditions and precautions.

Mobile *Svedana* box. Treatment during *Pancakarma*, Society of Friends, Berlin, 2018, photo credit: the author.

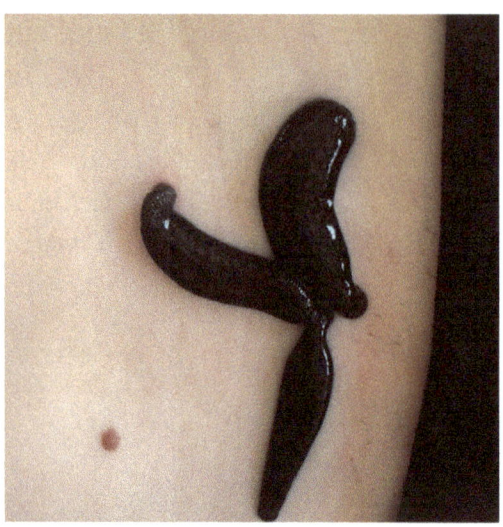

Raktamokshana at Society of Friends, Berlin. 2020, photo credit: the author

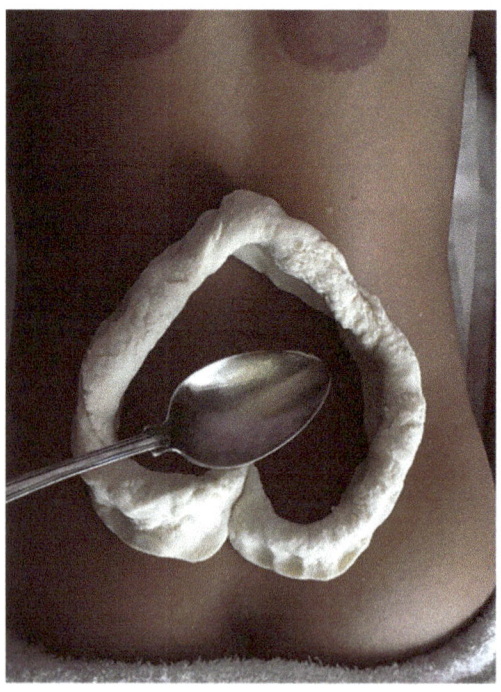

Basti with *Mahanarayana Taila* during *Pancakarma* treatment (big blue dots are from cupping) in a case of slip disc, IBS and chronic pain syndrome. 2018, photo credit: the author

Footnote: the transcription of *Pancakarma* might vary from author to author from *Pancakarma, pancakarma, panca karma, panc karma*, etc.

Experiences From Society of Friends, Berlin on the Application of Shirodhara For Patients Suffering From PTSD

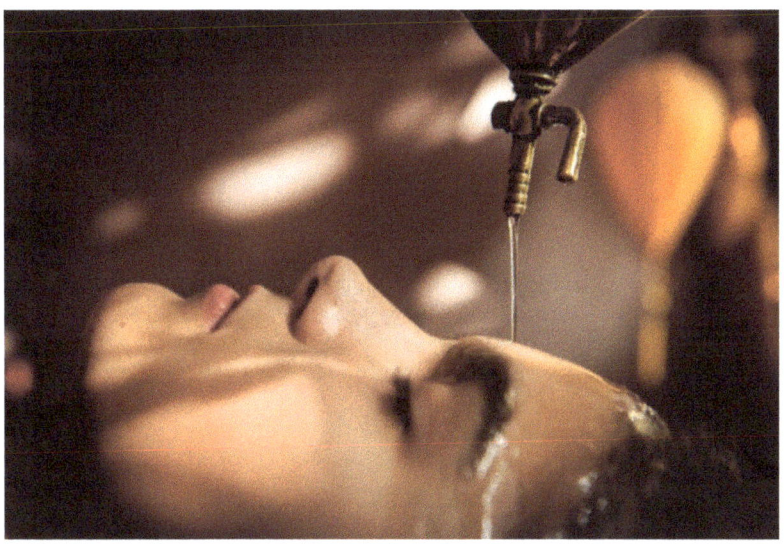

Photo: the author. A patient is undergoing *Shirodhara*, Olation of the forehead, as part of the treatment plan. Society of friends, Berlin, 2019

Shirodhara is a highly refined treatment against *Cittodvega* (anxiety, neurosis) and *Unmada*. However, during the treatments, staff members at Society of Friends observed randomly the opposite effect to the planned one several times.

Patients got into severe anxiety attacks, started breathing chaotically, crying or reported an increase of sleeplessness. It was like looking down into a dark place, some said.

Therefore, I decided to find the cause of such dramatic feelings and unpleasant reactions to a method that proves hundreds of years' experience wrong. Could this really be the case?

However, we discovered quite quickly whenever I was in the treatment room with my staff and the patient; the patients settled emotionally quite fast. It seemed the trust they had in me was one of the most significant aspects. We managed to install a feeling of safety when I stayed in the room for a little while and then left when the treatment was up and running but informed the patient with a goodbye that I was leaving now.

Looking into the setting of a *Shirodhara* from the perspective of a traumatised patient, a lot of the unexplainable reactions made sense:

- The patient is alone in a room with a practitioner they probably have not seen before.
- The patient cannot see the therapist as for *Shirodhara,* the therapist stands behind the head of the patient.
- During the treatment, the eyes and ears of the patient are blocked with cotton buds.
- The blocked senses make it difficult to trust.
- They can't reassure themselves that the situation is safe as they cannot move or see anything.
- The patient receives a treatment that can result in a passive drunken state of mind.
- The patient cannot move in this state or escape to a safe place.
- The procedure might be new and the treatment involves sensations on the head and skin.
- The patient is in a completely quiet room that can cause a feeling of isolation—knowing that no one might come in and check on them for some time.
- After the *Shirodhara* treatment, the patient is left alone in the dark, with eye pads and mostly cotton earplugs, lying down for an unknown period.
- The patient is unaware of the sudden interruption of the dark and quiet space by removing the cotton buds and pads.

The above observations led to assumptions about what type of trauma patients will most likely respond with an adverse effect. Women suffered the most, particularly when they had experienced their trauma in the form of child abuse.

In the majority, those patients had experienced the abuser coming into the room at night, when they were asleep and helpless. Memories came back, memories of the hyperalert state as soon as the darkness comes. Moments of uncertainty, not being able to escape to a safe place, being alone with a person, unable to control the situation, etc., led to a necessary change in the layout of the treatment.

Shirodhara is one of the most impressive ayurveda treatments for trauma, with quite a limited number of applications (mostly ten in a row, but sometimes only three are enough). Therefore, the modifications should be the ideal way to treat them minorly, but to the point.

Other patients had been victims of knife attacks that happened unexpectedly in the dark, from behind, without warning. The introduction to darkness as a safe place is the biggest problem we have had to face.

Modifications to the treatment with *Shirodhara* for traumatised patients

We took a lot of care to create a safe space for the patients once we had figured out where the problems came from. We are now seeing the all patients days in advance of the treatment and they need to be seen by a knowledgeable ayurveda practitioner or doctor. Likewise, the practitioner should introduce the patient before the procedures to the whole staff and all details of the treatment.

Unlike social media and advertisement suggest, *Shirodhara* is not a wellness treatment. The application of *Shirodhara* is a method to re-connect with oneself and soothe the troubled mind and the anxious heart.

To establish a positive physical and mental response pattern, repetition of any treatment is necessary, this is even more true for *Shirodhara*. Relaxation needs training and the procedures should be repeated several times until one can really see the manifestation of a change in response and behaviour. We aim for 10% in the first weeks. Therefore, the patient starts treatment well prior to the *Shirodhara* which involve deep relaxation methods.

Society of Friends, Berlin encouraged the patients to do "homework" where they observed their breath-hold, tried meditation or had other straightforward tasks to perform, which gave them structure and a sense of self-care under supervision.

Some of these exercises included daily reports of BP, pulse rate and other vital parameters which can be easily uploaded with a standard Android or iPhone.

For patients suffering from PTSD symptoms, a safe space is crucial before the treatment of *Shirodhara* begins.

Once the patient and therapist decide that they are ready and faithful to explore the *Shirodhara* effects, a plan of preferably ten treatments in a row is needed. Achieving the desired effect requires the patient to be treated at least once a week, preferably twice. If *Shirodhara* is performed in the busy centres of European cities, patients often cannot come in more than once a week. This is considered as the minimum number of treatments per week. Gaps between more than one-week treatments require a new set of treatments, starting again with number one from our experiences.

In a retreat centre or during intensive programs like *Panchakarma,* daily application recommended can be performed for better results.

In the days of no treatment, the patient receives homework of self-inspection, self-care, breathing methods or other techniques to keep the thread of treatments uninterrupted.

Society of Friends, Berlin, initially started with the traditional one-hour treatments. The effect on the patients turned out to be too intense in many ways.

The patients experienced post-*Shirodhara*:

—nausea

—dropping of BP of more than 40 mm/hg

—an increase in heartbeat rate

—hallucinations and

—numbness.

The patients were not allowed to go home on their own, drive a car, cycle or use public transport. For safety reasons, they had to be silently accompanied by a close friend or relative. From this experience Society of Friends, Berlin decided to cut down the application time and encouraged the patients to wait until they fully recovered from the treatment.

Between every ten to twenty minutes, the BP and pulse rate were checked and patients were closely monitored. When left alone in the entrance hall, they often reported anxiety due to the deep relaxation. Sometimes hunger occurred due to parasympathetic stimulation and small sugary snacks were provided for comfort. The idea that a good friend should be silently waiting with the patient and then accompanying them silently home turned out to be the best setting.

Unexpectedly, most patients were able to find someone happy to help. As traumatised patients often feel alone and not able to stay in close contact with friends, a surprising observation was made:

Those friends who were asked to pick up the patient reported:

"I was relieved that now something good is happening," "I was happy that finally, I knew how I can help," "Usually they refuse all help as interference and now I can give support, which makes me feel better," " I can see that someone understands their situation, takes care and I can be part of it," and so on.

Besides the help of friends, reduced treatment times were offered and adapted after each session. If the patient was fine, healthy and relaxed, one could start with ten minutes application, followed by five to seven minutes resting time while lying down and another half an hour in a sitting position. Healthy for *Shirodhara* means, in particular, there should be no *kapha* related diseases of the head, like sinus problems, phlegm or *pitta*-related problems like migraines, inflammation, etc. In general, all head conditions described in Shalakyatantra are exceptions and *Shirodhara* should not apply in any of these cases.

Symptoms of *Shirodhara* Unwanted Effects in Traumatised Patients According to Observation at Society of Friends, Berlin

Some patients, particularly those who have not experienced a safe place recently, reacted with arousal, a state of sudden onset of anxiety, increased heartbeat rate, flashbacks and often freeze symptoms or hyperventilation. Instead of experiencing deep relaxation, they were overwhelmed with stress symptoms like:

- Arousal (60 %) (all *doshas*, yet the reaction to the arousal depends on the *dosha*).
- The blood pressure could rise to 220/160 or (10%) (more likely *pitta* patients.
- Drop to 78/56 (30 %) (*kapha* and *vata* patients.
- Sudden big gaps of more than 40 mm Hg like 180/80. (20 % of the patients) (*vata* Patients).
- Hyperventilation (5%) (*vata* patients.
- Flashbacks (10 %) (*pitta*/*vata* patients.
- Freeze symptoms (15%) (*kapha* Patients.
- Insomnia after the treatment (30%) *vata* and *pitta* patients.
- Headaches (25%) all *doshas*, depending on location and quality of pain.

Therefore, it is recommended to check the BP each time before and after the application of *Shirodhara* and the pulse rate.

An unstable pulse rate is a sign of aggravated *vata*; if the acceleration is dominant, *pitta* also increases.

If the pulse rate or/ and breath rate increases during the procedure, *Shirodhara* should be stopped immediately.

Interrupting *Shirodhara* for Safety Reasons

The therapist explained to the patient in a calm, focused and stress-free manner that the *Shirodhara* would pause and for their safety, they had to follow closely all directions .

Kapalabhati Pranayama was performed to counteract occurring hyperventilation breathing patterns. The practitioner had to remain calm and was asked to immediately direct other staff members to help the patient into a secured body position (sitting up).

Staying close to the patient during their arousal, removing all equipment that might block the senses, such as eye pads, ear cotton buds, etc. and helping the patient sit up and breathe calmly and slowly, focusing on exhalation were the required actions.

Distraction is helpful as well as reality checks:

—orientation of the patient
—name,
—date,
—time,
—continuing a conversation that started earlier.

Daylight usually helped calm down the patient, so curtains were opened immediately.

Tea was provided. Conversations about what happened were avoided until the patient wanted to share the moment, ask questions or reflect calmly on the experienced feelings.

If the patient felt steady, calm and centred again, the practitioner sometimes offered another round, however shorter oil dripping, while leaving the ears open.

Some patients were able to address what caused the distress and the therapist could ask for specific ideas on how they could feel safer or more comfortable.

A patient who had been in a situation where they could not escape might have re-experienced helplessness in the case of sedating and calming procedures.

Like any other deep relaxation method that is hypnotising (inducing nystagmus), *Shirodhara* often leaves patients with feelings of immobility while feeling exposed. Patients reported that they felt as if they could not move their arms, legs, head or speak. A sensation of heavy eyelids might have occurred, too and triggered a feeling of being stuck or at a dangerous place that was unexplainable.

The above observations on patients with PTSD happen to less than 5% of the general patients with no PTSD. Therefore, most therapists will probably never come across this situation. However, it still should be part of their education in *Shirodhara* thought to be prepared, warned and know how to handle it lovingly and professionally. In the case of trauma and PTDS, the therapist will most likely come across these arousals in at least every second patient.

According to the research done at Society of Friends, Berlin, it is strongly recommended not to work alone with traumatised patients with intense methods like *Shirodhara* or *Pranayama* but have somebody around to help in case of any crisis.

If the patient is unable to attend the sessions regularly (lack of money, time, difficulties in organising pick up, etc.), they can be taught to imitate the movement of olation process. Simply the action of a finger dipped in oil and then writing on the forehead in the same left-to-right manner, with the same movements.

Of course, the effect reduces, but the patient is enabled to reproduce at least a part of the effect of *Shirodhara* and might integrate this in their daily life routine or any sudden case of distress. This substituting procedure is only effective if the patient works with an ayurveda therapist and their brain and body are already familiar with the expected feelings.

I tried to dismantle the complex procedures of ayurveda treatments to the core, like *Shirodhara*, to reduce the costs and make them affordable and accessible if the patient could not come in often enough for a continuity treatment.

My question was: What is possible to reduce, still achieving the best results?

To abide by the rules set down by ayurveda's greatest thinker and physician, *Charaka*, the patients should not start any treatment process that they cannot afford to complete. I tried to break down the approach to the essentials to target the needs of each patient and therefore make the treatments affordable and accessible by reducing everything to the necessary. It starts with small things that in the end cause a difference in price altogether:

Patients are requested to bring their own oil (saves me time to order, carry, buy)

They take it home after the treatment, boil and filter it at least 3 times. (they are part of the procedure, are aware of the costs and production process, we do not need a storage place or expensive oil collection).

They bring their own towels and sheets (saves money for laundry, replacing sheets and towels on a regular base).

They bring their own tea and refreshments (self-care learning, no staff needed for kitchen work).

Just these measures alone reduced the costs around 40 eu/treatment!

The process breaks down into treatments that are cheaper, safer, still efficient and more accessible for the individual patient. Starting from bringing their oil and towels, which created awareness, responsibility and a feeling of community support, the patients became part of a more significant project. They were contributing to the education of apprentices and junior students. As apprentices and junior students were interns and did not have to pay for their specialisation education, working in this framework led to efficient and cheaper treatments "for all" and "at any time."

These changes from exclusive setups in spas to rear medical procedures performed similarly in India resulted in the growing number of patients in general and PTSD/PTS patients in particular. The studies are based on hundreds of cases of successful treatments at my place, Society of Friends, Berlin, over more than 35 years.

Check List from Society of Friends, Berlin:
How to Perform *Shirodhara* Safely for PTDS and Trauma Patients

A safe, quiet and warm space will be the perfect condition to let go and experience.

Music or smell might help the patient feel that they enter a different space altogether where everything done is to comfort and protect them from all outside worries.

Check the pulse and blood pressure. Blood pressure can drop or increase in relaxation time, so they might need to stay on for a little while after the procedure until the BP is normal.

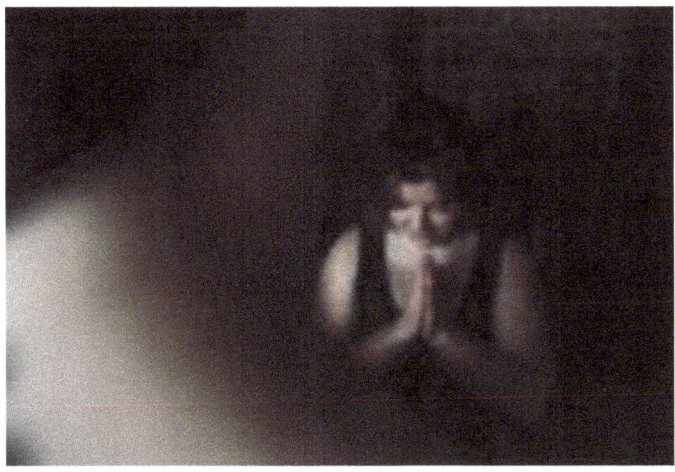

Photo credit: Anastasia Shchedrina. 2020

1. Check the room temperature. It should be fresh air, but not chilly.
2. Prepare yourself: let go of all worries, anger, stress.
3. Wash your hands in a gentle ritual.
4. Warm up the oil, best in the same room so you can watch the temperature at all times.
5. Set up the table: you need.
   a towel on the table, large.
   smaller towel under the neck.
   a large towel to cover the body, so it does not touch the blankets.
   Under—mattress heating.
   olation tool for the massage table at hand.
   the pot should be clean and shiny at all times.
   A big bowl for collecting the oil.
   paper towels.
   2-3 blankets.

Indian mini—brief if needed.

6. Clean all the surfaces before you start the procedure.
7. Wash your hands again.
8. Welcome the patient with a cup of relaxing tea. Make sure you have enough time even when the patient arrives late.
9. Make them feel comfortable, safe and relaxed at all times.
10. Allow the patient to change privately; a privacy screen is helpful.
11. Avoid too much talking about the day's activities; instead, suggest a 5-minute meditation together.
12. Once the patient is in the right mindset, allow them to rest on the massage table.
13. Drape the blankets around them in a caring and attentive, loving way.
14. Start with a gentle neck and shoulder massage with fragrant dosha type oil (15 minutes) or even with a full body massage, abhyanga style.
15. Continue with a gentle face and ear massage.
16. Take your time to connect.
17. Check the oil temperature; it should be above blood temperature but not hot or cool (only in high pitta conditions do we use **tarka**, (buttermilk churned with water.
18. Prepare the patient's face: put cotton pads over the eyes, soak in rosewater, plug the ears with oiled cotton buds, cover the eyebrows with cotton wool strings.
19. Cover the shoulders with pre-warmed towels.
20. Check first if the oil is running smoothly. Have a second vessel at hand.
21. Start in the middle of the forehead.
22. Complete the turn of the eight, up and down, as slow as you can; follow the movement with your eyes and circle around three, out to in, in to out. You should be able to follow the direction of their eyes under the cotton eye pads. They should move close to the centre of the eyes, not too far sideways or inwards. The eyes will follow the movement for a while. If the hair is thick and long, the oil might collect in there, gently repetitively squeeze it out.
23. According to the dosha condition, Citta and daytime pour the oil between 10-50 minutes. Keep the temperature steady.
24. Make sure that you can be comfortable for the entire time; the best is a sitting position.

25. Once you have finished, breathe.
26. Then wring the patient's hair gently but firmly to remove excess oil; repeat this several times with a gentle pull to activate the energy centre.
27. Gently dry rub the oil from the shoulders.
28. Be careful not to let tools drop or drip oil and avoid noises.
29. Wrap their hair with a towel.
30. Allow them some time to rest, but not more than five to ten minutes or the blood pressure might drop, drowsiness or an increase in kapha in the head can occur.
31. Make sure they are kept warm at all times.
32. Help them to sit up, slowly, mindfully, caring.
33. Offer a tea while she is sitting up.
34. Observe her condition; they should be stable, not nauseous, alert, but relaxed, not panicking. Avoid telephones or any other sound-making electronic devices in the room.
35. Make sure they get picked up minimum after half an hour. Have a cosy waiting space prepared.
36. After each patient, it is essential to clean everything thoroughly. The vessels need special attention. They are sacred vessels. Clean with fat-removing soap and then rinse with hot or even boiling water. Watch your hands. You are removing mental and emotional impurities together with the sticky oil. Make sure to clean the tube.

    Once you have finished all patients for the day, allow the vessel to soak and rest in boiling water for at least fifteen minutes while you clean the room. Open the windows. Move your body, release tension. You have shared a deep inner space with someone else. Clean yourself with cool water before going home.

Conclusion

Shirodhara could help the traumatised patient experience an extraordinary relaxation without feeling helpless or vulnerable. However, in the beginning, a safe space needs to be created.

Trust and precise guidance are essential figures in the success of the treatment.

Shirodhara can help traumatised patients get in control of their heartbeat rate, normalise their breathing patterns and even strengthen the ability to fall asleep. It is a method that should be incorporated into all PTSD programs.

Shirodhara has significantly helped and supported my patients who struggled with drug addiction and withdrawal symptoms. As much as withdrawal symptoms subsided, the patients—unexpectedly—stopped craving. The general idea that the addict has to suffer through withdrawal to understand "the mistake that they are making by self-harming" is replaced with the encounter of being loved, held and sheltered.

If addiction is considered an adaption to a traumatic injury, condemning the victim and exposing them to even more suffering could explain the high rate of failure of rehab therapy. It could also demonstrate that the addiction disappears if the underlying pain of rejection, abuse and unsafety is removed.

"Why are people taking cocaine, crystal meth, alcohol? These are pain killers. So, we have to stop asking: why the addiction? We have to ask: why the pain?"

(Gabor Mate, TED Talk, The Power of Addiction, The Addiction to Power, seen 5.10.2020)

Mate emphasises and so do I, that therapists should undergo specific psychological training to discover PTSD patients early and efficiently handle arousals. Markus Ludwig, Midgard Kalari, Ayurvedic Education Centre, Germany, collected *Shirodhara*-related problems in patients decades ago and I was fortunate to hear from those patients directly. It was the first call that I received that *Shirdodhara is not just something ready—to—go* with everybody. Unfortunately, his project came to an early end as networking between therapists at this early time of ayurveda in Germany (1998) was not yet existing.

Western psychological approaches towards trauma and PTSD are relatively new, as the term "trauma" was introduced to psychiatry only forty years ago. Modern therapies are getting refined, adapted and developed. They are, however, much different from one another in treatment methods and analysis.

However, a fundamental weakness in all of these approaches reviewed in this thesis is that Western Trauma therapy is either primarily analytical and focuses on the traumatic injury itself or it does on the adaption of the particular patient. Therefore, it is not a synthetical approach, meaning it is not embedded into a multidimensional holistic concept of belief, nor it is embedded in a concept of a general responsibility of society, country, family and friends.

The therapeutic methods of western trauma therapy are often not adapted to the diverse backgrounds of the victims nor the diversity of mental, emotional, psychological traumatic responses. An often desperately needed combination treatment on physical trauma alongside with a treatment of psychological trauma. The focus of trauma research in the west from its very beginning was on American soldiers, mostly Vietnam veterans and later Iraq and Afghanistan veterans.

Their experiences led—in my eyes—to a too early conclusion which implemented that trauma could be standardised with a particular outcome and probably even a similar later-on perspective. It did not pay attention to the continuity of daily traumas, generally higher in number, experiencing domestic violence, violence against women, LGBTs or POC and child abuse patients.

Misinterpreting trauma as an individual's faith and not taking responsibility and action for changing socio-psychological measures and procedures will not generate trauma. POCs or LGTBs claim that the "white men's" therapy does not respect their background and does not consider their constant psychological stress from dysfunctional racist and bigots societies.

Ayurveda instead provides a comprehensive, complete lay-out of long-term tried, tested and approved therapy guidelines over thousands of years. From spiritual rituals to healthy eating, from self-massage to intense therapeutic practices like *Pancakarma*. Ayurveda structures daily life as well as the sickness in life. Through understanding connection, society, self and improving mental and physical well-being, Ayurveda establishes a safe space for the patient. It is a multidimensional concept of self-enhancement, self-care, responsibility for society, the environment, the welfare of others.

Ayurveda provides and encourages experiences as well as it demands obedience to rules. Taking responsibility is one of the key factors for the patient's self-support. There is always a free choice. Free choice is an essential paradigm as it offers the patients an opportunity to grow at their own pace. Enforcement limits the patients' curiosity for recovery as enforcement can produce resistance, replacing overall sensitive guidance.

The Ayurveda therapist, the *Vaidya*, has numerous tools to treat patients individually and precisely according to their needs while embracing the difficulties. It thrives from various minerals and healing herbs to medicated oils, from breathing to milky baths, from mantras to physical exercise, each of the methods customised to the individual patient, the age, the season, the problem, etc. the stamina, the moon and the stars.

The patient's global and individual meanings shatter during a traumatising event and even worse through continuity of assaults, pain and discrimination. To enable the individual to contribute to society and family in the best possible way, they must consider unique and global purpose as understanding oneself in a safe and supportive place. Contributing to community and family means the basic needs are fulfilled without denying food, water, housing and the supporting the right to safety and education.

Each individual is born with an urge to discover their purpose and explore their possibilities and borders—this is considered the satisfying meaning-making needed to live a fulfilled life. As trauma can also be passed on over generations like war traumas and the Holocaust as the most studied examples, understanding the global and individual meaning and how to restore it is essential to create a safe space that can generate healing.

Ayurveda helps the victim and gives clear measures to improve life at all measures to prevent illness by leading a happy and balanced lifestyle. Developing or reconstructing global and individual meaning is essential for recovery and healing. Ayurveda and yoga can provide and rebuild the feeling of safety and pleasure, care and meaning.

A Priori Beliefs and Meaning

A-priori-beliefs in the world, in contrast to the mixed blessing of self-enhancement or repressive coping, a more broadly adaptive component of resilience is favourable. It is important to understand resilience. Some people suffer less from traumatic injuries and events than others. Those who suffer less believe in a generalised conception in life by the conception of life as justice, fair, predictable and "good."

However, for others, traumatic experiences can shatter beliefs and leave the patients vulnerable. The experience has changed the perception of some individuals that the world is a hostile, random and dangerous place.

A related construct to a priori-beliefs is *meaning-making*. Park (2010) proposed that an important distinction is between the effort to find a meaning (meaning-making efforts) versus arriving at a meaning ("meaning-made").

Self – Views

Self-improvement as a way of healing is not embedded in a concept. However, we see more and more self-empowerment courses pop up with no concept whatsoever, but mixed, fusion concepts that waver between goddesses and self-exploitation by favouring forgiveness to the perpetrator as the way to heal.

Often victims end up in cults or even, because they do lack the red flag security guard, get into new traumatising sexual assault with the personal of those "healers".as long as the victim on the recovery trail it is so important to have guidelines, supervision of us therapists, security by the law and many more helplines along the way.

Therefore, I emphasise continuing studies on the treatment of traumatised patients with ayurveda and yoga. The specific, individualised, adapted and constantly redirected treatments have enabled patients to step out of the dominance of psychiatric intervention and medication. An economic outcome of treatments with ayurveda might be positive and the patients have a high success rate in going back to their lives and contributing to society.

The long-term trials and empiric studies that I was lucky enough to conduct, strengthened my belief and hope. It turned into an absolute conviction that trauma therapy has to be integrated into ayurveda in modern terms and studies and not ayurveda into trauma therapy. Trauma therapy is already an established figure in ayurveda for thousands of years, but it is helpful to learn from modern approaches and evaluate them. Ayurveda provides a transparent evaluation system, whereby I am humble to publish my attempts here for the first time.

4.   The Case Studies: The Heart

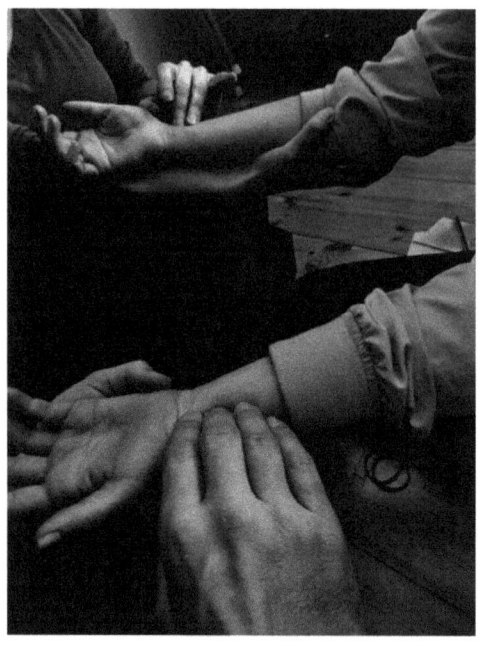

Photo: the author, students learn pulse diagnosis during an Ayurveda Yoga *Chikitsa* Training in Berlin, Society of Friends. 2018

Conclusion of The Case Studies

The case studies written pay my respect and display thankfulness to my friends and patients. They do not, however, display only success. They do not show an easy, happy road after having received treatment. They are raw and even uncomfortable to read. Still, I consider them as material from where hopefully others will head off into a more refined and individually tailored plan right from the beginning. My research is embedded in these case studies and some progress is seen. They are important in order to encourage the therapist, *Vaidya* or medical doctor to create their very own adaptions and research themes.

Faith is important, courage and fearlessness in the research of trauma. It is worth every minute.

The most meaningful example for overcoming trauma in an ayurvedically based way means embedding it into a social quest of support, family support, financial support, not questioning the victim and meaningful daily self-practice is *Kapil*. They are an example of resilience that came from support towards recovery. During the interview, he recently told me that he had seen the movie "Hotel Mumbai," which depicts the terror attacks personally but primarily invented personalities. I felt my hair rise. He said: "Well done, a lot of suspense in the movie!."

While working with refugees from Syria during a project for the European Union, I designed for *Massage, Meditation and Mindfulness*. I observed something so touching and powerful that I felt again my thesis supported: By being in a situation where the teacher had asked the participants to imagine a safe place, a home, one young woman from Damascus broke out in tears.

None of the Syrian women was going and patting her on the shoulder, trying to minimise her grief by goodwill and well-meant suggestions. They all went closer to her—bit by bit. Closer, in deep silence. Some of them were crying soundlessly, too. They showed a genuine, innocent understanding because they managed to stay in touch with their own feelings. They were not afraid to face their grief, losses, sadness.

This silent companionship, the support without adding interpretations, accepting the patients' trauma as a part of their narrative and recreating safety and self-care are the most potent tools we also observed during our clinical trials. Teaching by example, says Mate.

However, the sad loss of Sueno highlighted that there are limitations as well We cannot arrange our own lives around an endless chain of patients in need, nor is it possible to cure everyone. That would be narcissistic and would only lead to manipulation.

Still, there are these moments when connection is felt by everyone working on the patient at this very minute. A connection that is not of the therapist and staff with the patient but a re-connection to the patient within themselves. The example of Amber and Greta are of such delicate subtleness. To understand that ayurveda and yoga incorporate a deep knowledge of the self that can be experienced and can change, therefore saving lives are seen in Amanda's case.

Trauma therapy should not try to absorb ayurvedic knowledge. How can such a complex holistic science fit into a specialised section without losing its true meaning, context and diagnostic tools. And, ayurvedic wisdom needs a better logistical and educational base when studied abroad, in particular to meet a traumatised self's exclusive and individual needs.

Ayurveda and yoga display already all-important measures, diagnostics and healing aspects. The west is asked to open up now and study diligently the depth of this science for recovery, resilience and healing of the traumatised self, traumatised societies and a peaceful world.

Studying the mind separately, Ram Manohar states—there is a risk of becoming mentally ill. He is convinced that one must have an enormous ability to love in order to heal the mind that is disturbed.

This implicates that therapists have to undergo self-practice and self-inspection. Ayurveda and yoga offer therapists practices to heal them before they inquire about the patient. The high standards of ayurveda and yoga education need to be respected and not watered down to consumable workshop format.

As an anxious species we are constantly stressed by not having control over our surroundings, emotions, but in connection and reconnection we can find ways to design a safe space and a chance to survive as species. As we desperately need not only more mental health specialists to fix the broken, but manage global destruction and fear related wrong doings from our politicians, global companies and all these people involved that live on our fear rather than creating connection and protection.

They say human nature is aggressive; they say human nature is competitive. It is just the opposite. Human nature is in fact cooperative, human nature is actually generous, human nature is actually community minded. *Mate, own transcript, 2012, The Power of Addiction, the Addiction to Power.*

The format of the case studies has been originally in 2 versions: one was in tables and one that is descriptive. For the book, I only kept the descriptive one to give an impression of the people, their life narrative, their attempts to heal and even our failure. The names are anonymised and replaced by utterly invented names, however the name of Kapil I decided to keep as the original one with his allowance.

We hope that through the research and the case studies from Society of Friends, Berlin, other therapists will learn and explore different ways how to treat patients with PTSD. The guidelines that were developed from the empiric experience, extracted in data, can become treatment guidelines in general for PTSD if more therapists contribute to their own research.

The patient, however, is introduced in a non-formal text as an individual person, rather than just a statistic figure.

The text highlights certain behavioural aspects, characteristics or habits that have been observed during the treatments and were of some importance for practical decision making. The second format is a very personal introduction to the individuality of the patients as well of their possible interaction with the staff of Society of Friends, Berlin. The case studies in this format are considered to be educational. They highlight the research measure, as well as the therapeutic standards at Society of Friends, Berlin.

Why was the descriptive format chosen? Whenever case studies are presented in medical research, there are mostly numbers and graphs displaying symptoms. Researchers have to standardise people's complaints, illnesses and diseases so that they can fit into tables and statistics and then finally the measurements themselves will become standardised and comparable to prove a case. The individual has disappeared. Pain, sorrow and joy, liveliness or suffering gets lost.

Without these qualities, empathy with the patients and their individual tragic life narratives is not possible. The view goes merely on results in percentages. This does not represent the healing aspect of the individual, their journey, their hopes and their set—backs until they finally might come out of this narrowed life path. This way, the reader is able to understand the complexity of each individual and treat them with the respect they deserve while reading their history.

Without the patient's trust in yoga and ayurveda and, last not least, in the practitioner or therapist, none of this research work would have been possible. Without the tremendous effort of the patients, their discipline and their struggle, none of the treatment plans would have come into life. It is through the patient's compliance, dialogue and discipline that the treatment plans and the knowledge behind them hopefully can change the life of others, too, who are suffering.

By asking my patients to use their biography and data for research and publishing purposes, I was unsure if I might indeed have crossed a line: a safety line created by trust that guaranteed protection in a life that is marked by vulnerability and shame, panic and often fear. This can potentially destroy the safe space created by the professional secrecy, which is guaranteed by law and an inner contract between the two parties in general.

The law guarantees that nothing bespoken will ever be reported to anyone outside the medical practice. By German law, therapists, apprentices and assistants have to keep this secrecy. However, my patients were mostly very enthusiastic that their narratives and treatment plans could change other people's life for the better. That their stories might be able to teach other therapists to understand, diagnose or treat better and save time that might get lost in wrong and insufficient approaches.

However, my patient's data is anonymised in order to provide protection. Medical researchers have to ask for permission, knowing that even the simple act of asking the question itself could destroy the subtle connection of trust between patient and therapist or even throw the patient back into painful memories and cause re-traumatisation.

The required permission was then given by my patients and thankfully I can publish their life stories of that tell us about the abuse that happened, neglect, violence, escape and finally their struggle for recovery. While keeping their identities anonymous, their case studies are published here.

There are no similar, equal, obvious or generally visible or clearly defined signs that allow the therapist to detect the patients suffering from trauma or PTSD easily. It can be crucial to know about their sufferings, their life in disguise or their experience of dangerous situations, their narratives of pain and struggles, adaption and despair. A medical practitioner must never judge their patients for their adaptations, such as addictions or for their often inexplicable difficult behaviour. Instead, all patients deserve compassion and professional help.

However, we know that a lot of us therapists have been struggling or are struggling with trauma. Often it is also part of our experience as therapists that by listening to the patients' life lines we can get badly affected, by being exposed to their sadness, grief or anger—and even sometimes, violence.

Every now and then, a patient might even overstep our boundaries, threaten us, trying to seduce us. Sometimes their stories might let us remember our own wounds. We might identify, overidentify, neglect and deny the patient's stories. It is important for us therapists to be open, to get supervision, to have support. Sometimes a patient's story might even sound less dramatic than our own or we even could envy their lifestyle, we have to discover where our boundaries are.

Some therapists in such courses that I lead, said: I have no boundaries. I am open. But, nevertheless, I do have healthy boundaries after all. I don't want to treat people who engage in sex with children. Or animals. I cannot relate. I am not covering up crimes. This is just an example but often we do not recognise our wounds that brought us into the field of healing in the first place and so we do not see our judgments, prejudging, anger or other emotional hinderance when we treat a patient.

It is an invitation to read the narratives of treatments of my patients. Each of them has an individual history not only before but also during their treatments. There were ups and downs, failure and success. Yet the majority of them were treated successfully over the years with our individually tailored treatment plans.

Understanding patients' narratives of their lifelines and that people are affected worldwide and every minute by traumatising events, it can become important to follow the wisdom of ayurveda and yoga and experience the difference of the holistic point of view. It can become important and helpful for the lives of the victims that we as therapists can see hope, meaning-making and the changes that are possible in order to try new-(old)ways.

Detailed personal case studies like the ones presented here, could help therapists studying how to detect the individuals' traumatic injury and see how and why their patient is suffering. They could even help to detect signs of trauma in a close friend. Long before any diagnosis could lead to treatment, reading case studies might help the reader to become perceptive to the secrets that so many people around us are carrying with them. Case studies in conjunction with the understanding of the values and virtues of ayurveda and yoga could empower therapists to provide individually tailored treatment and support.

Again, I wish that my great thankfulness towards my patients will be reflected in the descriptive personal case studies. I take them back into the light, as they are not just numbers and casualties. With their courage, openness and support, they contributed to helping others.

Sueno

Sueno is dead. He ended his life at the age of 37. He was my student at the Academy of Natural Healing Arts, Berlin, for many years. His dream (sueno: Spanish translation for dream) was to become a healer. Coming from a broken world, he had all the intention to heal others and though healing himself in an ideal world. In my memory, he was a slender, good looking man with a broad smile when he came in to work with me or be the patient.

His family came from Bosnia during the Yugoslavian war. They arrived as war refugees in Germany and lived in a sporting hall for a couple of months together with hundreds of other war refugees camping on the floor. His father was a drunkard, abusive and left the family when they needed protection most.

His mother was schizophrenic, helpless and abandoned him in his childhood, often for days and even weeks. She was neglecting his needs, particularly for shelter, warmth and food. Her abusive words hurt him deeply but he had decided to go through this challenge. Finally, he saw her painfully suffocating in her death and made peace with her. Already at the age of 7, Sueno was diagnosed with multiple personality disorder as well and received medication. Unfortunately, there is no record of the medicine that he had taken.

From his childhood towards his adolescence, he just had a foggy memory of taking drugs, house squatting and parties until he found people who offered him a safe place.

He moved in with them to one of Berlin's squatted areas, living in a trailer without running water or heating but with people around him who listened to him and loved him. His new friends often shared a similar past, so understanding was there as well as violence at times when they could not figure out what was a reaction to a present situation or a dark memory that invaded the current moment. They ended up cursing and shouting at him.

2 weeks after his mother's death, he was diagnosed with late testicular cancer. His wish to live and heal was shattered again. He lost ground. His multiple personality disorder episodes were increasing. He himself tried to anchor these people inside him but the images were overwhelming. Before the cancer diagnosis, he used to come once or twice a week to my clinic for either a treatment or an internship. Now his life was falling to pieces. He was not afraid of death. But his will to live was broken.

He stopped the clinic's internship, but came in for daily treatment. We applied Shirodhara to help him sleep and breathing softly as nervousness and anxiety were moving from his heart to his head. He received regularly Pranayama *Brhmhari* to connect lovingly with himself.

Then he could not even handle the treatments anymore as his schizophrenic episodes lasted longer and longer and dissociation at times did not allow him to follow any instruction safely. His usual soft and gentle voice (K) changed to a brittle voice (V) or even to a harsh (P) tone. He was afraid he could injure us when anger and the feeling of being lost would take over. Being treated well and loved was difficult for him to handle at those times.

He was instructed to inform us at any time if something was going out of control. Through breath awareness, he felt he was capable in telling mood changes early enough to find a safe solution.

From the moment I turned the keys to open the door, Sueno was there till I closed down. 13-15 hours a day he sat on the couch, seeing people coming and going. He took some *Jatamamsi churna* in combination with *Tagara* churna in boiled in milk, altered at times with *Ashvagandha* churna and *Brahmivati*. He inhaled camphor when he felt he was about to lose contact with the world around him.

Slowly, by and by, he felt hours of relief and allowed himself to receive gently *padabhyanga*. He said he felt like living in a glass bowl, where there are terrifying enormous bats coming to drink his blood. He mentioned that when he smelled the ayurvedic oils and herbs that we used in the clinic, a feeling of wholeness and holiness spread and he felt relieved.

I then had to go on a study trip to India.

We made an agreement in the form of a contract that he would not kill himself. He was aware that he still needed constant supervision and care at this time of slow recovery. After a consultation with an ayurvedic doctor I received an email from him and his hospital, saying "dogs that bark don't bite", informing me that there was no danger at all that Sueno would commit suicide.

Sueno was devastated. We tried another allopathic hospital. They took him in for 2 days. The national insurance refused payment, stating that he had received treatment from his childhood onwards with no proper improvement and therefor they stop all payment for further medication or hospital care.

I was in India when I received the phone call from his boyfriend, telling me that they found him dead after 2 days, in the bathtub. In the letter Sueno left behind, he apologised to me that he broke the contract.

Sam

Sam did not come on her own accord to see me. The first time she was sent to see us, the social worker had set up the appointment. For my security, it was explained, a trained Dobermann dog came along with the social worker, making sure that Sam would not attack me.

Sam was a young woman in her late 20s, victim of street violence and emotional abuse from her early childhood on. She had suffered from some recent injuries like a broken arm and wounds as she was a trainee in an Integrative Social Institute to become a carpenter, yet got in trouble with the boss and finally destroyed most of the furniture including the doors of the institute.

She was told I would be the chance to avoid a criminal court case if she behaves well. The whole situation was not very promising, as there was no anamnestic file to understand what might trigger her outbursts of anger and violence.

As I could not spend the time with the social worker and my patient threatened by a dog, I sent dog and social worker off and asked them to return in one hour. Spending some time alone with Sam built up trust between us, when she then felt that I was not afraid and she was not the "monster", not the "wild animal" as she was described by the social worker.

Communication was very difficult as she seemed not to have learned much to feel or express herself or had given the space and the time to talk to herself. So, I finally decided to take her to the yoga room. Practical appliance of yoga is always the best way to remove doubt.

She was wearing jeans and a Canadian woolly shirt and did not want to remove her socks. Her expression of shame did not really fit into the fear of the social worker that she might get violent, yet I felt we carefully had to draw lines and move rather slow so she could feel safe.

We started in Tadasana, the simple standing position. For someone practicing yoga the first time, it is usually a bit dull, as one feels: oh, I did this before, waiting at the traffic light.

With Sam, it was different. Slowly and mindfully, the voice of my assistant Romi lead her into the pose. Starting from creating awareness into her toes, sole of the feet, ankles, calves, she realised how her breath changed and that she actually had to struggle hard to stand still. It took her a while to understand that she could also end the pose. She was so absorbed in the voice and counting of the breaths that she forgot that she was actually just standing yet experiencing something new and interesting.

She had to learn that she was guided into the pose but it was fully her own decision to end it at any time. The aim was to regain control over her life by slowly practicing it on the mat. She also realised that from the moments, when all thoughts and emotions flooded into her mind, the observation of the breathing introduced her to a focused stream of thoughts—even if these thoughts were merely about how to get out of that pose. She then got picked up on time and promised me to come back.

The social worker made compliments that my furniture was still intact. I felt bewildered.

A week later Sam came back. This time we decided immediately to send the social worker straight into the park and Sam looked like a child that had been playing a mischievous trick. She herself went straight into the room, where there were still other people from the previous session. She ignored the fact and sat down.

She said, "Last time it was boring. I don't know what this is about. Why should I focus on my toes?"

Besides the feeling that we might lose the subtle connection, I realised that she actually went into a dialogue. A dialogue with herself (boring) as with me, criticising me and expressing what she wanted. I asked her if she is ready then to take a challenge and she said yes.

So, we chose Vriksasana, the tree pose. She totally hated it. She was struggling and dropping and getting angry. So, we provided the wall for a feeling of stabilisation and security and she succeeded easily in the pose, although she kept on blaming herself as she thought she had cheated to get there.

So we emphasised now on leaving the wall by bringing awareness back to the toes and she understood that we were actually introducing her to stabilise herself through breath and awareness. We worked with Sam quite regularly, the occasional interruptions happened when she delivered herself to the emergency room because of suicidal attempts.

Slowly, she allowed us to touch her.

We started with a foot massage. My assistant started a gentle massage while I was sitting next to her. Allowing us to do so was another big step for her.

She allowed herself to be appreciated and valued by others. She could respond to care.

By and by, she included the oil foot massage into a day program for herself. She said she felt different with it.

Her suspicion disappeared very, very slowly but a feeling of confidence and of being at a good place established in her.

Each time we saw her we were happy that she was still alive as well we wondered what would be the next step on her journey.

One day my daughter brought a little bunny to the clinic, that was abandoned by its mother and we brought it up with a syringe, getting up every night 4 times just to feed it. It survived. Sam saw the bunny and wanted to hold it. We all stopped breathing when it sat on her hand and snuggled into her fingers. My daughter did not know about Sam and had given that tiny bunny to Sam with so much trust.

Sam took a deep breath. She asked: "Can I keep it?"

That was more than we ever expected. She felt ready to look after a helpless being! Not only that she had established some yoga routine and included her favourite oil foot massage, she felt stable enough to look after that little bunny, a helpless, defenceless creature.

There was a gentleness in her that we all could not believe.

We never knew what had happened to her in her life. But we could see and feel that yoga and ayurveda brought her to a safer place.

I stayed in touch with Sam for several years. She sometimes came along when her new work schedule allowed her to take a day off. The social worker and the dog were fading memories of the past.

She started cooking and established more self-care moments. She built up friendships with colleges and was able to address her positive feelings.

One day, she came to the clinic in tears. She asked if we could take the bunny back. Besides all the progress she made, the suicidal attempts persisted and increased in November that year it got worse as it was dark and rainy. Her food choices then got messed up as she felt she lost ground and she walked straight into a vicious circle.

She said it got too stressful as she went to the psychiatric ambulance in the night but had to be back till bunny wakes up because she did not want him to be alone in the mornings, finding out that she was not there.

We are still in contact and we all know that there will be times of a relieved mental state, but there will be also times when everything goes downhill again. Ayurveda and yoga provide the tools to get back on track. It starts with the toes. It starts with the positive memory of self—care. That the road to the better life is seen again.

Greta

Greta came to my clinic on recommendation of several of her artist friends in Berlin whom I treated. Her friends told her: "Don't expect anything. We cannot predict what Manuela will be doing. Just go and see her, you won't get what you want anyhow!"

So, there she was. Open-minded but tremendously sad and depressed, suffering from hay fever and asthma. She had moved from Austria to Berlin years ago but still her voice and way of speaking was Austrian, a comforting singing sound.

Her health issues were treated previously successfully in Vienna with acupuncture and herbal medicine. So we decided to start from where the positive experience was, where she felt comfortable the most.

Her body was round and soft, her big brown eyes always a bit sad and her thick brown hair surrounded her with no chance of keeping it tidy. She herself admitted that being messy in general was a big problem in her life. She said the pain that she went through as a child of an always drunken mother that even forgot to feed her child left her in a position where she gets lost and dissociates from everything around her. She thinks this dates back to when she was a small child and the police found her at times being alone and hungry on the streets of Vienna.

Her grandmother, who herself was in a dysfunctional relationship with the grandfather, looked after her but unemotionally. She then was sent off to her uncle, where she was more or less the maid and was lectured every day about his Nazi ideology. She never received protection or loving care in her early years.

Greta began to resist. She went off to Vienna, became a teacher and an artist. On the outside, it appeared as she was about to make it, as if the shadows of the past were fading and in fact even had made her stronger. But then again and again, people let her down, betrayal and threat for her bravery got in the way.

Each time, she needed more help to get onto her feet again. Each time the problems got bigger and something of her strength and stamina, together with her endurance and resilience, got lost. However, her tremendous kindness and helpfulness remained.

When we started the treatment with acupuncture and ayurveda herbs, she was happy. The results were promising. She also enjoyed the food routine and loved to cook.

But then her life got out of that fine balance. It drastically changed from being in an interesting job (although her boss was bullying her) at the university to finding herself suddenly unemployed and broke. Greta's life has always been that of a ship in rough storms with the Capitan hoping for the best but not having a map at all.

In Greta's life, there was one unforeseen challenge overlapping the other. She lost the work she was good at. She did fundamental work for Holocaust survivors and was active in all kinds of political anti-right wing action groups.

243

But she was completely broke and had to rent out her apartment and did not know where to sleep herself. She stood up for democratic rights and spoke up against fascism but she was threatened by anonymous stalkers.

She did great work as a critical historian, but the stories of the people who did not survive the Holocaust were engraved in her memory. She was on stage as an opera singer but the opera had only one performance. Each time, she had to pick herself up and think of what to do next. Suffering from PTSD often stopped her creativity and talent as an artist and locked her in for weeks.

She had spent all her money after she had lost her job—but she created a wonderful project: because she loved the clinic and its people lots as it had become a steady place in her life, she invented "The Ayur-Wiener Film Salon". Struggling again with major depression at the time, she still managed to set up the place, chose a film and cook an ayurvedic meal for the audience. I was so moved by her, she was so inspiring.

Her ideas were big but not too far from becoming real. Greta was not a dreamer but a practical and caring woman.

When her depression though was increasing the asthma again and the asthma increased the depression and there was no money, she came in every Monday evening for treatment, cooking a meal for all the people still working there and for our last patients.

It was mostly the first meal that we all had during a busy day. Her way of caring for us was never intrusive or manipulating. It was a clear support after clear observation. Her ideas reflected a spiritual way of her chosen background as a Tibetan Buddhist. The intensity of how she cared about was loving and supported by her meaning making. It never was mothering or disrespectful.

She was surrounded by friends. But Greta got hurt and hurt again by the work and living circumstances she was in.

Her intimate relationships, though, turned out traumatic. Each time she broke through the thin ice and was about to drown, we went into new intense treatment phases.

In Greta's treatment, I left the pure path of ayurveda. After she had several Major Depression episodes, I agreed to her therapist's prescription of SSRA. The dosage though was increased every couple of weeks, turning Greta's active and beautiful spirit into a numb and uninspired functioning tool.

We then slowly reduced the dosage again and when the psychiatrist realised as well that her symptoms were worsening under increasing medication he agreed to supervise the reduction (I had done this with other patients on these drugs—under close supervision of their psychiatrists). She lost weight and felt emotionally lighter, too. Yet, the ups and downs of daily life she felt she could not handle without getting to sleep better. And the anti—depressants had helped. We then tried different herbs but sleep remained a big problem.

She practised yoga and breathing exercises on her own and we saw her almost every week for massage and acupuncture.

She was an exceptionally good cook and so I hired her for Pancakarma. She was fully dedicated—and then collapsed. Her motivation was so high, but her expectations of her as well—

In the last year when I was away most of the time, we developed a treatment plan with herbs and female hormones to treat the peri-menopausal symptoms that increased the depression, the sleeplessness and night sweats. It worked out quite promising—before she was betrayed and let down again in the very moment; she felt she could be happy and could finally experience to trust. That promise was broken. Her heart almost broke.

She still is fearless but she lost hope. She speaks up but for others and she will try to find her own voice to speak up for herself.

She looks after others but hardly allowed herself to feel good. She hides, she disappears, she loves, she suffers.

But with the spiritual insights, the techniques of ayurveda and yoga and the company of her close friends, she will stand up again. As she finds meaning in her life by understanding the cycles of life, understanding the function of the mind, cherishes the food. She also knows it is practice.

Treatment plan:
Dravyaguna:
The general description
Mustha 1/4Tsp—1/4 Tsp—1/4 Tsp with honey water Shatavari 3 caps—3 caps—3 caps
Guduci 1/4 Tsp-1/4 Tsp—1/4 Tsp in milk
Bala 1-5 tablespoons in emergencies, boiled in milk
Occasionally Jatamansi (as it is under worldwide conservation, we had only very little left to use!) as ghrtam
Acupuncture: Manaka acupuncture treatment, 10 golden needles and other formulas

yoga and pranayama Shirodhara, etc.

Kapil

Kapil is a gentle speaking man with perfect manners and appearance. He is slim, in his 50ies, wearing a perfectly tailored suit and always a winning, generous smile. His eyes are steady, his voice is clear and the way he talks is pleasing and comforting. He is kind and welcoming, his shop as an open door at all times. He is funny and honest. His story is a very special one as it shows different cultural aspects in the aftercare of traumatised patients as well as self—healing and supportive methods to overcome PTS.

It was a day that throw the world into a shock. Unbelievable pictures were shown in the news: Mumbai was under attack, the *Taj Mahal Hotel* was in the centre of a war from an Islamist group named Laschkar-e Taiba with just 10 attackers arriving from Pakistan in a tiny boat against a city and it' s lifestyle, statement and money, leaving 174 people dead and hundreds injured, an uncountable number of traumatised victims, observers and helpers.

Every day the world was horrified and we were breathlessly watching the news. Frozen by the idea that people are fighting for their lives for hours after hours and finally for even 4 days with no break at all.

However, now, the *Taj* has been beautifully rebuilt, there is always the shadow of the attack felt in the building. It is present in the big memorial stone near the entrance and the lounge for all the victims, on the guided tours through the building, the rooms, the endless corridors, the lounges.

I met Kapil in his sparkling jeweller's shop in the basement of the *Taj*. We spend the afternoon with him, my assistant Romi and I, drinking chai, eating with him, singing. At some point, he started telling us his story of his survival of the four devastating days:

For the full 4 days of the attack, he was lying on the floor, not moving at all. He showed us the place. He showed us the places where the bullets hit the wall—they are still in the wall, covered up with some plastic. Proudly he pointed towards an enormous jade carved Ganesha statue sitting on a shelf. Kapil said, he will never sell the statue, as it is a lifesaver.

He removed the statue from its spot—and behind it, touching the statue, a bullet was pointing into the shop. We did not know what to say. While he spoke, the horror was present and we were silent, but our hearts were screaming. As if the walls would echo every second, he had to live through. Echoes of the fear, echoes of the detonations, the shots, the screaming.

Every year since then I return to the *Taj*, speaking to Kapil, spending time with him, talking, listening and enjoying his clear presence. Every day, Kapil repeats a sacred mission: he sits every morning in meditation at 04:30 AM in Vipassana meditation for 2 hours. As often as possible, he meets his master in meditation for joining inspirational talks and full day Vipassana gatherings or retreats. Silently observing his breath, full of utter awareness to all the subtle changes in his consciousness and the body.

After the meditation, he types into his phone whatever had influenced him, what he experienced in the meditation or what he felt the world should know and sends it off via "WhatsApp" to his more than 600 friends all over the world, including Romi and myself. Every day, he makes sure with his "WhatsApp" that we know he is there. That he is safe. He is not silenced to survive anymore. He is speaking up, he is showing his presence.

He influenced me and my work a lot with his way of coping with his traumatic experiences. He became a key figure by looking into different ways to deal with profound traumatising events in life. He also introduced us to another meaningful difference to most of my patients: the *Ta* was paying their staff. They did not have to fight in court cases lawsuits they would not win.

In Germany, after the Christmas market attacks, the first information was that each individual had to apply for compensation from the attacker himself (who was shot, however) or his family (KriPoz,5/2020). In the west, we carefully try to reintroduce people to the surrounding where they had experienced the shock of an attack. The Berlin Christmas market was even considered to be shut down.

The survivors of the Christmas Market attack were invited to be guided after more than a year to visit the location, not at Christmas time however, briefly in the presence of a psychiatrist. The survivors of the *Taj* attacks instead are different in so many ways. They all came back as soon as their wounds were healed and continued working there. No avoidance of places, smells, moments, time, memory days.

In fact, there was a big party held, where all the survivors from all over the world were invited to participate and celebrate life. In Berlin, candles are flickering in memories. At the *Taj*, people are looking into the future. In Berlin and Paris, the places of remembrance are now majorly secured by electronic gates and armed forces, they are massively secured to enter. At the *Taj*, the entrance is secured with guards and electronic handbag control but not to the degree that one actually would feel trapped—because one can leave through all the side exits at any time.

India is a country that is known for mental peace, yoga and contemplation as well for its battling with poverty, hunger and terrorism. The courage and bravery of the survivors of the *Taj* are an example of how community, social support and connection can help to heal traumatic injuries. Creating a supportive environment of people as well as financial aid, inner survival and finally recovery can be possible, as seen in the example of Kapil.

The skills that Kapil brought with him were those of contemplation and awareness, of focussing on the moment. Tools that help him day by days to return to the moment of NOW. Having a supportive family who understands is the other pillar. As he said in the interview: " I learned that every single moment is unique. Moments of sadness are there and moments of happiness. They all pass."

The presence of peaceful mind at every moment is hard to achieve. When a person gets traumatised, the present can become a constant threat, it is filled with memories with no exit door. In Kapil's case, he chooses the practise of the awareness of the present to experience the world from moment to moment—as new as possible.

The tools of awareness and meditation are a perfect rope that hold him. No avoidance. Everything in his life, every experience and now even the lockdown because of Covid-19 in Mumbai, is a tool that he enjoys in order to master his wandering mind. The attacks became the biggest challenge in his life. However, he learned to accept this challenge and embrace it and became an inspiration to others and showed me a key tool for treating traumatised patients with a new confidence.

Using pranayama and practising awareness and mindfulness on a daily base is a key tool to cope with traumatic experience and its arousals, best to be embedded in a safe, caring and supportive surrounding and a caring society.

Samuel

Samuel came to my clinic with every intention not to listen to whatever I would say. He had seen "too many quacks before", he pointed out as a welcome, yet his assistant had insisted that he should give it a go. He was working on a project in Berlin which had directly followed another project before, this one without any recovery time. He has had no time off since 8 months, just a weekend here and there which he used for intense partying to "let some steam off".

A normal workday was around 12—14 hours of concentrated but often chaotic work schedules and conditions. Poor food, irregular working hours, including night shifts on a constant change, described his days.

His appearance was somehow exceptional, even in our place. His voice was deep, warm but a bit too loud, his body overweight, wearing a colourful shirt, colourful scarf, a lot of rings and bracelets, he was definitely doing well on being right in the centre of everybody's attention.

A peacock almost within our small place. He was polite, charming and flirting with my staff. It is a quite common behaviour for men we see in the clinic, which makes it difficult to continue a proper investigation. Men sometimes stay in a flirt mode to avoid proper answers and it can become tricky to get to the core of the problem. However, he was very open to our questions. In fact, he discovered the anamnestic questions as entertaining and he received a lot of attention.

Samuel told us that he was sent to see me because he had become "a pain in the ass" to his staff mostly due to his intense pain, followed by his self—medication with codeine, ibuprofen, alcohol and drugs.

Samuel told us that he started working in the entertainment industry at the early age of 17 years, developing an intense lifestyle of having plenty of money to spend—followed by times with no work, no money and selling whatever he owned.

I simply hoped that he will leave as soon as possible as I did not feel prepared to deal with his massive pain syndrome neither his drug abuse, while working under horrendous circumstances.

What could ayurveda possibly do for him?

He explained that he suffered simply from continuous neck pain. Looking at the neck, long red scars were seen and he explained that a physiotherapist broke his vertebras once in a session. The communication resembled a Russian doll investigation.

We started with the information: neck pain, moved on to damage of the cervical spine caused by a forceful and bad intervention by a physiotherapist. Continuing to investigate how the primary injury happened we found out that he demonstrated risky behaviour while hang gliding where he had the initial crash, breaking his arm and causing damage to the vertebras. Immediately after the accident, he went back to work and even right after the surgery, he had no resting time.

He told us the story of injuries, pain and bad treatments with a bright smile, as if he had done something mischievous or even funny.

He got a bit more trustful during the first examination as he realised that I did not offer a cure. He said he had heard from everybody he saw for treatment before me: "yes, no problem, I can cure that".

I, instead, openly said I do not think that I can cure his pain. His life/work circumstances cannot be changed, so I don't think what I have to offer would work. The long working hours, lack of sleep, high blood pressure and poor diet with obesity alone were enough to treat under "normal" circumstances. He got frustrated and upset and insisted that he want to try his best. The change of attitude was stunning.

So we opened the next Russian doll: drug abuse. At the time he came to see me he had created a self-treatment plan: Codeine drops, more than 15 /daily Ibuprofen, Nurofen, Aspirin etc more than 1000mg /daily In combination with Vodka and other spirits Daily consumption of 2 bottles of wine Weekly consumption of cocaine, more than 2-3 gr each day Smoking cigarettes, a package a day. Other recreational drugs like Ecstasy, MDMA, crack cocaine occasionally. Sleeping pills: Valium, Tomazepan, Zolpidem.

As I am a health practitioner with a healthy lifestyle, I have had no idea what these drugs are, what kind of physical, emotional or behavioural response they cause. Only after detailed information seeking it was clear that they had a strong wake up effect on the nervous system, a hyper-alert state, paired with the need to move or talk for hours, but in combination with alcohol or Valium the previous drugs were antagonised and a dulling effect becomes dominant. And they all, including the alcohol, are pain killers.

Most of my patients are actually in a so-called poly toxic self-treatment situation. As I mentioned earlier, poly—toxicity is not the exception but mostly the "normal". However, the other big group of my clientele were yoga teachers or yoga students, so they tried to cope with their traumatised self in other adaptive ways. With the research of Gabor Mate, we learnt to ask the question: what does the patient gain from it? Why the addiction? Instead of shaming-blaming the addict.

The combination with alcohol ("downer") allowed him to modify the push ("upper") effect of the drugs. So there was kind of "balance" between hyperactivity and dullness achieved.

Having a closer look into the nature of most the consumed drugs one can understand, most of them are painkillers, including the alcohol. Following a theory presented by Gabor Mate, PhD, that drug abuse and addiction are actually a way to try and soothe the pain. So, we have to look deeper into the pain Samuel is suffering from. He mentioned that he started drinking as well as using recreational drugs at the age of 16.

Coming from an artistic family of painters, Samuel found himself always under the pressure of competition. He still feels that all family members have been much more talented than he is. Even various award winning in his artistic specialty cannot help the feeling of worthlessness and heal the lack of self-esteem—

In his early ages, the family was moving throughout the world following the jobs of his father. There was no steady home, no continuity of time, culture, language, schooling. Growing up in northern Europe, then moving to Arabic countries finally he found himself in a boarding school, accompanied by his disliked elder brother.

He tried to escape the boarding school several times, was punished and put into detention until he finally was thrown out of school. His beloved and adored father died unexpected the same year and left him unprepared for whât was coming. His mother developed a rare form of Parkinson's disease with Lewis bodies in the brain and spend her last years in psychiatric hospitals until he finally had to stop the machines.

At this point, I felt that the Russian doll was growing bigger and bigger and my hands were empty to deal with all his pain. However, there was the determination that he made all the way here and I should do something—now!

I think I hardly ever felt so powerless.

I started an acupuncture treatment to work on the pain but he complained that he did not like the pain of the needles. The steam bath, *svedana*, after *snehana* ended in a panic attack. The oiling was horrible for him as he was covered in sweat already before the *pinda svedana* was even applied. Frustrated I offered some yoga, absolutely convinced that he would leave in a hurry, but no, he stayed.

We started with simply yoga therapy: leaning his back against the wall, feet apart and front (*Utkatasana*). He was advised to lift his arms over his head and try to touch the wall behind him with extended arms. He could not manage this at all: he was able to lift in a 60 degree, his left arm 80 degrees. We then tried inner rotation with bend arms, using his exhalation to contract his perineum (*Mula Bandha*), his throat (*Udhyana Bandha*) and using his diaphragm to maintain the action (*Jalandhara Bandha*) of his arms and back.

Followed by a prescription of *Mahayogarajaguggulu*, *Brahma Vati* and *Haritaki,* he was sent home. We all felt exhausted.

We tried to have regular follow-ups as he called the next day, reporting a significant decrease of his neck pain! I was more than surprised as we know now that the constant use and abuse of pain killers causes often enough the pain memory in the brain which is harder to cure than any pain itself. The brain repeats the pain pattern often without the cause or trigger.

Luckily, his body reacted so well. After 3 weeks of cancellations, last-minute appointments at 11 PM and other obstacles, we decided to perform *rakta mokshana* on the scar tissue, using 3 leeches.

We had to stop the procedure due to heavy bleeding, panic attacks and general discomfort while trying to keep the position steady so the leeches would not drop off. The bleeding continued for more than 8 hours after an early removal of the leeches, but the stiffened tissue softened and allowed us to increase the challenge of orderly movement in the shoulder girdle. Shirodhara and full body oil dripping were accepted by Samuel, helped reducing nervous tension and promoted relaxation.

As it was Samuel's first contact with ayurveda and yoga, we were surprised how quickly he responded to the methods as well to the medications—besides telling us all the time that he did not think that any of this helps at all. After 3 weeks, he stopped most of his self-prescribed pain killers.

Surprisingly, he continued his daily regimen of yoga therapy in the morning. Samuel integrated some suggestions into his daily life, like a change of diet and to keep his bowel in order: *Haritaki.* Every weekend was a challenge, as the behavioural pattern of indulging was stronger than all ideas of ayurveda.

For some time, Samuel received weekly *Abhyanga.* He felt the best of the treatment was the routine and the feeling of some order and direction in his daily life of constant changes and overworking. He still hated the yoga exercises, describing them as torturous—yet he felt that they had a positive effect on his body and so he kept on practising regularly. Samuel enhanced his daily practise on weekends or time off with a strong workout on his rowing machine.

To support impaired liver function, we prescribed *Liv 52, 2 times 2* from Himalaya Herbals. From time to time, we used *Aroghyavardhini* to promote bowel movement and liver function. The Aroghyavardhini reduced his reoccurring fevers as well.

After all, the whole setting of ayurveda treatment and care, he described as warm as a motherly hug.

The care and attention he received, as well as the honest interest in him as a person, was creating an atmosphere of trust and openness. He was not the famous patient with bags of money. In fact, he complained that we were too cheap for the effort we had put into treating him. Respect you cannot buy. For some patients, it feels too cheap and they leave. Some patients can simply just afford our treatments. As I learned in my first lectures with Prof N.S. Gupta ji from Nadiad, Gujarat, that according to Charaka, we are not allowed to treat the poor patient.

After years of an inner struggle with this sentence from Charaka, I decided to follow my own interpretation. Of course, we cannot start treating a patient and finding out later that he cannot afford the payment, we would have to interrupt the treatment, causing probably more damage as if we better would have never started. But there are ways to finance in many other ways—For richer patients there is always the donation option for social projects.

In the case of Samuel, the money discussion was an important part of the treatment. As it helped him to understand that we were not the slightest interested in his money or fame he felt acknowledged as a person, as an individual, treated with all the respect that any other patient received.

In Samuel, we saw a strong Pitta-Kapha condition. Stamina, a lot of physical power and endurance, to take on the most difficult jobs as a challenge. Being an artist that requires a lot of handy man work as well as creating designs, it is a Vata as well as a Kapha requiring work. Creating objects, designs and then staying on for long hours is very demanding.

He loves to collect art, objects and prefers a life in the garden, surrounded by friends (Kapha)—while often following the call of drugs, party and night life (Pitta). He suffers from depressive episodes (Vata Kapha). When he entered a room, he was shining and all attention turned onto him (Pitta) which was counteracted by his feeling of shyness and insecurity (Vata) Over the years, insecurity grew with severe traumatic incidents accidents, robbery and mobbing.

What he learned in the time of treatment was to remember his life's goals, creating a safe space and holding on to a daily routine. Even if Samuel often fails to maintain the routine, it is there in his head and whenever he feels everything is falling out of his hand; the pressure is becoming too much, pain and depression are drawing him into a self—damaging behaviour he feels he can find a hook to hold onto.

Recovery and addiction are the 2 poles that mark his life and take up a lot of his time. But with yoga and ayurveda, he found a meaning making a third way of acceptance and hope.

Amber

When Amber came to see first me, she introduced herself with a gorgeous, winning smile. She was looking so cheerful and stunning, a professional dancer, Mediterranean, winning everybody's heart immediately.

She had asked for an appointment as her sleep was bad and she truly needed help as she was travelling a lot through time zones and could not get enough rest. She mentioned some back pain, too, that kept on bothering her for a while.

She looked and sounded calm, speaking with a gentle soft voice, patiently trying to find the right words in English. By the looks of it, she appeared to be in balance, happy and cheerful. We did the Ahara/Vihara List discussion as usual; I checked the tongue and pulse. The pulse was feeble, superficial in all parameters, thin and sharp, her tongue had a bright red tip which in Oriental medicine we consider as emotional stress.

Her eating habits were far more conscious than those of most of the dancers I usually saw. She had a nourishing breakfast of cooked vegetables and rice, which she enjoyed, normally a good and satisfying vegetarian lunch and dinner, no particular allergies.

There were no eating disorders in her history. During dance performances she skipped meals and ate late but returned to a good routine immediately afterwards.

The only thing to mention, really, she insisted, was her lack of sleep, mainly the inability to fall asleep. As treating sleeping disorders with patients who are travelling overseas is always a trial I decided to start with the physical examination of her back pain and see how she reacts to ayurveda massages that might calm the mind, too.

As she lifted her shirt, I was struck by what I saw. Her whole body was stitched up with 17 large scars from a knife attack. The scars were close to her heart, on the side of her neck, above and into the kidney region, on the full left side of her lungs. The performed operations left her with 5-7 cm long, swollen, red scars all over her body.

As she did not say anything, I decided to give her more time until she might build up trust and felt to give an explanation. The scars widely blocked the muscles from normal functioning. The restrictions of the myofascial tissue must have been painful, yet she spent the days with intense physical exercise of stretching her tissues.

We decided to start with Abhyanga with medicated oil, Mahanarayana Taila and Pizhilli, pinda svedana, straight after the Abhyanga. She said she felt some kind of beautiful energy passing through the scarred tissues. As if they are getting back into life, as if they are coming back to the body. We continued the treatment for several days. She said she had a significant improvement in her body work, all tissues felt fluid again. The Mahanarayana Taila is not only an oil against pain, injuries and scars. It is a three dosha oil.

The Mahanarayana Taila that I am using in the clinic originates from Shri Ganga Pharmacy, Rishikesh. It contains quite a bit of Camphor which is proven by my patients to be helpful in the case of emotional arousal to centre and ground them quickly.

She also said that she felt more relaxed after the oil appliance, as if she was held and kept comfortable.

We decided to continue the massages for another week and we observed that her whole body was feeling open and heavier, rooted, resting on the warm massage table, comforted by the gentle strokes, repeatedly administered from right to left, left to right.

After this time, she decided to open up and bring up again the subject of sleeping problems. Amber revealed a horrifying story of her life where her ex—boyfriend attacked her on her way home. He stabbed her in the back, continued with absolute cruelty on her chest and throat, determined to destroy her, to kill her. She remembered that she reached out for help, that she saw neighbours that closed the windows when she screamed for help.

At the time the ambulance arrived, she was passing out. One first aid helper continuously said: "don' t sleep, when you fall asleep you die". Amber then told me, each night, when she tries to fall asleep, she hears the voice: "Don t sleep—" then, at this point, her breathing would change and she has to jump up.

So, we decided to try pranayama in a supine position. We both tried carefully to create a setup in which she felt comfortable and safe and at the same time could carefully and controlled remember her daily night terrors in order to learn to manage them. Amber had already brought some yoga practice with her and fortunately, her body awareness was subtle and trained.

So we build up several bolsters against a wall, so that the ground was stable, yet soft and she could remain in a fairly seated position.

We then tried to breathe our way through any change of the breathing pattern, re-directing awareness into distant parts of the body.

Pranayama Treatment
We started with exhalation 6 Inhalation 4
Then ex: 8 Kumbhala 2 In 6 Kumbhaka2
She did this as a regular daily homework.
Ayurvedic Herbs
We tried several combinations. As with many trauma patients, she reacted badly to calming herbs like Brahmi, but was far better off with simply Ashvagandha.

She took Ashvagandha, 2-2-2, regularly for a short while but we all felt that she responded to pranayama so well that we did not continue the medication.

Yet the oil application was needed to be continued in order to stabilise the emotional factors and the Vata in Hrdya (the heart).

Arousal Control

Each time Amber and I met, we lowered the supporting bolsters until she was able to lie on her back on the floor without re-living the horror of the attack. While lowering, we thoughtfully created awareness into the feet, rotating the thighs out so she had to actively stabilise her core. Her sleep was improving by and by, as she kept a steady routine of pranayama and yoga. The fear of going to bad slowly vanished.

At times it came back, yet she took it as a sign to deepen the practice. She left for a longer stay in an ashram somewhere in Kerala, lived a month in a jungle.

We tried to stay in touch loosely over the following years so I always knew where she was. She became a yoga Teacher out of her own dedicated and honest practice. Her way of restoring her moment—to—moment awareness and growing into an experienced practitioner was amazing.

As part of my exploration for this work, I finally called her. Amber was very touched when I explained to her how ground breaking our meetings had been. Since our very first meeting, almost 10 years had passed. She explained that since the day we met, she kept her pranayama practice as it felt good and she could see the progress so clearly. She said that every morning she sits down for meditation. Sometimes good, sometimes bad. Amber said: every day there is something different. But she continues.

She was happy to tell more about her life, being a sexually abused and neglected child, that she had reached out for help before the knife attack happened but no one listened to her, no one believed her.

She said it was a relief that I did not ask anything about herself, her past, her injuries when we started. She said the absence of intrusive questions gave her the feeling that she did not need to explain and from there, re-live her trauma. Not asking means not explaining from her side. It created a safe space for security of non—judgement.

Till nowadays we have to live with the fact that in case of attacks and rapes, of violence against women, that they are not heard by the police, by court, that they are not understood and most of them keeping quiet. Even in court cases we see that women are not believed or they are even been told that they are as well responsible for what has happened by being with the wrong people, wearing the wrong clothes, saying the wrong things.

After several intense treatment weeks, Amber was on a good way. By observing and listening to her body, we found a way to put her back onto her feet. Awareness and subtleness through ayurveda and yoga had unfolded their soothing, healing powers. Pain relief translates as emotional release, as tension increases pain. Amber felt softness and kindness, acceptance and care. She discovered something inside her that wanted to live, that wanted to feel whole and nourished again.

She told me that she was not free from the frightening memories. But that she now could live with them. They come and with them there are moments of despair, doubt and depression, but the good moments are there, too. The good moments come from an increased self-care. They come from acceptance. They come from the pacifying breathing, the herbs and the field of ayurvedic healing that never leaves somebody once one got really touched by it.

When I met Amber, there was not much research on trauma published. There was not much on treatment published either. Mostly the recommended treatment as a Gold Standard consisted of psycho pharmaceuticals like Haldol, Valium or Tavor to control anxiety, panic attacks and depression. A lot of the patients, though, including Amber, refused to take these as they felt cut off from their real selves.

So when I started the treatment with Amber, we both walked into a completely unknown field. Thanks to her open-mindedness, her body awareness and her trust she was the first person that received an ayurveda yoga treatment after surviving the worst, long before treatments in the west with Trauma yoga were advised.

Her deep understanding of the effects of yoga and pranayama on the scattered mind was the key. Ayurveda, with its nourishing applications, it is an amazing treasure of herbal medicine opened her heart.

Ayurvedic diagnosis:

She had Pitta dominance with Vata in her Prakriti as well as in her Vikriti, here to mention the increase of Vata at her heart.

Gunas: Rajas, disturbance of *Nidra* (anidra roga—diagnosis of sleeplessness)
Mamsa dhatu affected, Asthi dhatu affected

Selma

Selma was brought into my clinic by one of my students, who was living next door. My student said that she had noticed that Selma has been found several times outside her home in a helpless state. She then became friends with Selma and observed more and more disturbing aspects of Selma's life that Selma considered as normal or even comfortable. In the beginning It took very long to set up any appointment with her as Selma was completely depending on the help of her mother, sister or my Student Natasha to leave her home.

Selma was shy when I saw her for the first time but friendly and open. She said she suffers from depression in the winter. That was all she found important to say. Her appearance was that of a young girl instead of a woman. Her round face with her dark eyes and wide-open forehead made her look appealing, sweet and charming. She dressed up carefully when she came to see me because it was a special event for her going out.

She did not feel much of physical or mental discomfort as she had locked everything inside herself. However, it led to a circle of avoidance that got tighter around her until she was about to suffocate in it.

The family fled the civil war in Yugoslavia and her first years in Germany were not bad at all. She went to a public school, learned German quickly, made friends and it felt almost like a normal life of a normal girl. Because she was not registered as a war refugee due to her Serbian national background, her legal status in Germany was insecure and she could be deported within 12 hours without warning. Her father got severely depressed over the times and when she was 16 years old, he hung himself. Leaving his family in despair and uncertainty.

She got married early but could not settle down in intimacy and found herself alone after a short time. Things got worse quickly from there on. While her elder sister seemed to manage everything well and effortless what Selma had ever wished for, like being independent, having a good marriage and 2 beautiful daughters. Selma felt being responsible for the happiness of her mother but could not even allow herself to be happy.

She tried to settle down and feel at home. But all attempts seemed to end in failure as her unsettled refugee situation reflected in the daily life in Germany. A hopeless circle: no search for an apartment could end successfully when it was unclear who would pay the rent, no job interview was doable without a proper visa which was depending on a job and the job on an apartment and so on. She had to renew her visa on a half year base, each time undergoing devaluating harsh inquisitions.

After being recognised as a trauma patient with the help of a report from my side she got One-Year-Visa which helped a bit to stabilise but still however, a safe space was not achieved for her. She started a 3 week education as an ayurvedic massager and for some time she was able to contribute to a spa place, filling it with her kind nature and softness. Yet when the dark thoughts and feelings and the lack of security hit her, she escaped into her shell life. She lost the job soon.

Selma was participating in our workshop for the European Union, which I started in order to help people with long-term unemployment and migration background to fill in their empty years out of work. It was a small group of 7 participants that she knew before from my practice and whom she really liked.

Carmen from Spain, a roman catholic, Masami from Japan, a Shinto believer, Romy, a Jewish Russian-Latvian, Magda, a Colombian catholic Yogini, Tidjan,

Voodoo believer from Martinique, Sue-Ellen from Brazil, an animist. She discovered the differences and the similarities. The other students also suffered from being displaced, having trouble with cultural understanding. They discovered their so different life stories in an alienated society and where surprised that each of them had a very different opinion about the goal of life.

We discussed the purpose of life because the workshop was about accompanying dying people. One should have an opinion, a purpose, a belief, because people will ask where they are going when they die. Selma shared a dramatic story with us about the Muslim Serbian funeral of her grandfather.

When she then heard the story of the Jewish funeral in Latvia, understanding that beliefs and customs can be in fact so different to what she took for granted. She said, writing it all down and then lecturing about it helped her so much getting back into these memories. Seeing everybody has losses, no need to bury everything in your heart and that there is compassion and understanding possible.

She helped the children's hospice enormously as her study on Muslim customs at death was very helpful to avoid mistakes in cultural cross overs. Selma discovered the richness of a culture that she carries. She started seeing that her way of relating to people, her generosity are key points of her culture and personal upbringing and that she in fact lives in so many values that she has not seen before.

During the workshop we practised breathing, pranayama, daily and meditative walks in the park, silent retreats and breath massage, Shiatsu and yoga. She realised how much she was capable with ease to feel the people' s tension, to be empathic and open.

The biggest experience from the workshop was that she discovered the healing potential of the work itself. By attending the workshop, she managed by and by to appear every day on the doorstep without excuses and mostly on her own. At the end of the day she needed a lift home because she felt exhausted but was proud of her skills. The skills were not only to help others but unfolded helping support for her, too, by diligently practicing them.

The setback happened after the workshop. But she did not give up, tried even to participate more into healing massages in the clinic, did pranayama teaching and enjoyed every time she massaged somebody or could help in the kitchen.

There were ons and offs. Sometimes she had to leave the room during a massage immediately or she did not turn up, sometimes she massaged until we had to stop her.

As she got better and emotionally more stable, her visa situation was still a big problem though, we lost a bit of contact. I see her life getting into an independence where she is trying to find her way, always knowing that ayurveda is there and we care.

Treatment: Pranayama and Dravyaguna:

shankhapushpi 1/2 Teaspoon, 1/2—1/2 boiled in milk

ashvagandha see dosage above

ahara vihara: self-care: self-abhyanga, cooking, walks she finally bought a dog who walks her.

David

David was ringing the doorbell as if we were all deaf. As he walked in, the floor was literally shaking. Although slender but muscular, he created noise wherever he was going, whatever he did.

As we had a lot of gentle breathing or Shirodhara treatments going on, we tried to get the noise under control. He apologised, while seconds later his phone rang loudly or he dropped his bag. He went back and forth while waiting, going downstairs to catch himself a coffee. Loudly he made compliments to my staff.

He was wearing a short, tight muscle shirt with Ganesha and OM on it, showing all his brightly coloured tattoos of fish and women on his well—built arms and neck. His hair was black and grey, slightly curly, thick and strong. Wearing a lot of Indian silver jewellery and Mala beads around his neck, he looked like what a western yoga teacher supposed to look like.

In my clinic, we used the kitchen as a place to have a pause, write invoices or eat.

It said PRIVATE in big letters on the door and the inside was covered with a bright red curtain. There was no stop for David! His head went in at all times, putting food, coffee and other things on our desk, asking for water or where to put his litter. His voice was loud at all times, slightly singing, not unpleasant, but felt almost substantially present. He said he had heard from other yoga teachers and students that I am an excellent therapist and I can cure everything.

By saying this, he already switched on the alarm system in my head. He told me that he is "the most successful Bikram Yoga Teacher in Germany", a style of sequences that are performed only at a very high room temperature.

In his first consultation, David was very excited and showing a constant smiley face. His smile stayed on even when he talked about his life's downsides.

David has worked all his life under tremendous stress through extremely high expectations of his family, who all were lawyers. His father died early at the age of 51 from a heart attack at work and David had to be responsible for his mother, who got severely depressed and unable to look after the younger children.

The family turned out being broke due to gambling of the father and they finally lost their home. The mother never recovered from the shock and stayed in a state of speechless amnesia.

David looked after her and managed to organise successfully the life for his siblings. Due to his capacity of planning and foreseeing he qualified himself as a management trainer but could not stop the attitude of planning and organising every aspect of his life which left him exhausted at the age of 25. He neglected his state and started to drink to be able to relax and finally sleep for 3 hours.

As the drinking and lack of sleep got in the way with his duties, he used cocaine, Ritalin and amphetamines during the day for almost 10 years. He said life felt like an ongoing party. Not until he collapsed on the street, causing a severe accident and harming others, he had any insight into his emotional structure.

Yet, after being hospitalised and undergoing psychotherapy, detoxing, he still carried the primary stress pattern, now transferred into his new duty as the best and most successful yoga teacher.

On this road to success, he lost his wife and family. They were disappointed that he did not share his emotions or his time with them and seemed to take them for granted. When they left, he did not really realise it until the letter from the lawyer arrived. He explained to me that in a state of higher mind, through yoga, one loss naturally the connection to the mundane world.

He had changed his diet after his stay in the psychiatric hospital, which he preferred to name a "retreat centre" from being a "monster meat eater" to "a wonderful sattvic yogi", now being on a diet that consisted only of raw food, absolutely no oil (because there a grain's pressed!) and pureed fruit pulp. He was completely vegan. Yet the amount of sugar in his diet in fruit juices and pulps was stunning.

He realised soon that by and by he developed a chronic rhinitis accompanied by an addiction to nasal drops containing ephedrine. As his condition worsened, the nasal drops were applied day and night, as he woke up during the night as he could not breathe.

During the day he took self—prescribed medicine, all rich in aromatic oils: orange oil, nasal drops, thyme and lavender capsules and thyme tea. His rooms were soaked with aromatic elixirs of all kinds. As we know from cross allergies, people who are suffering from an allergy to early blossom like hazelnut and birch, are mostly suffering from cross allergies:

Strawberries, apples, carrots, oranges, mandarin, celery, kitchen herbs: thyme, basil, sage, majoran, peppermint, spearmint, lavender, soya and all its products, hazelnut, all other nuts (that includes strawberries and blueberries), mustard, dried peas.

That basically was a clear reflection of his diet. People who suffer from allergies should avoid raw foods completely, particularly fruit. Nuts are full of fungus, which is contributing to allergies, as well as they are high in cross-allergic potential. So I had to convince him to try a completely different diet, where everything is cooked and prepared in ghee.

He believed that all the symptoms he suffered from where actually detoxing symptoms and that he was on a very special way of cleaning his vessels and his body on his steady way climbing towards enlightenment. It took him weeks to come back and not until that he slowly realised that he had to change. His stomach was gurgling at all times, he had big smelly stools and constant smelly gas trouble with cramps, burping, diarrhoea and constipation, irritable bowel syndrome and the list could go on.

We agreed to a 3-week trial of change. I offered being karmic responsible for the ghee consumption (he insisted on this bit). His symptoms of chronic rhinitis and digestive problems vanished very quickly with the change of diet and additional pippali that he decided to follow further ayurvedic treatments to deal with his losses and his denial of sadness. Receiving his first ever abhyanga left him in tears. He continued his treatments with abhyanga and additional pranayama on a regular base until he left Berlin to spend time in India for further studies.

His changes were massive. He became soft and gentle. We often had to look for him as he got quieter and quieter. It was a pleasant, respectful, successful work after a pretty wild start.

In my presentation in Nadiad, International Conference on *Shalakyatantra* (diseases of the head) on ayurveda, Gujarat, India 2.-3. September 2016) I presented my research on CRS in trauma patients. Traumatic injuries seem to be often connected to CRS (Publication on 2nd International Conference on

Salakyatantra, Mahagujarat medical Society, J. S. Ayurveda Mahavidyalaya and P.D. Patel Ayurveda Hospital, page 95-100).

One part of its aetiology is the change of the breathing pattern through the nostrils during stress. The nasal breathing becomes sharp and therefore starts irritating the mucous membranes, causing cracking, infections and swelling. Additionally, the application of harmful substances like nasal drops and often cocaine are contributing to the problem. As David showed a very good compliance, we could close his case as a happy one.

Treatment:

Nadi Shodhana morning and evening, extending the exhalation phase up to double the inhalation

Dravya:

Triphala churna, 1-1-1

Tagara 1-0-1

Shankha Pushbi 1-0-1 in milk

Anu thailam morning and before leaving the house, alternately Ghee in the nostrils

Olation of the ears

Shirodhara weekly for 6 weeks, later Shirobasti

Steven

Steven, a 27 years old student of economy, lived in both Paris and Berlin when he came to the clinic for a little check—up. He loved to travel and to live in several places and countries, not being anywhere for long. Steven showed up at the clinic on the suggestion of his best friends. They were tired of hearing him complaining about his wheezing and shortness of breath, his tiredness and lack of motivation.

He was pleasant to look at, neatly dressed, his clothes carefully chosen. He looked a bit too elegant compared to his Berghain clubbing friends. He actually looked overly concerned about his appearance and style. He spoke with a soft and gentle voice, a lot of the times I had to interrupt him because I could not hear clearly what he said.

He had a history of CRS for 14 years already with previous treatments. Mostly he received antibiotics at least 4 times a year for a minimum of 10 days, Cortisone Nasal Spray, Asthma Spray with endorphin and cortisone and emergency shots in case of acute status asthmatics. He reported being a heavy smoker since the age of 13 (25-40 cigarettes daily) and did this with an apologising smile. He said it helps him coping with his hay fever that he suffered from almost all year long now but it got worse in Berlin (the city of Berlin is covered up 47% with forests and parks).

He was actually not too concerned about his lung problem as he said, he was so used to it and also, he failed to stop smoking so many times that he thought, obviously his body needs it. Not being able to support his health by a very rational decision, we were not sure what we actually then should responsibly treat. He decided, therefore, that he would much prefer to be treated for his atopic dermatitis.

He said the rough patches look like a contagious disease and so he really got concerned about it as it inferred with his dating life. It destroyed the cashmere jumpers as well. (V)

Due to his asthma, he has not done any sports ever. To stay in shape, he had decided to put himself on a low-calorie diet. While he thought that he probably lacks nutrients, Steven took a vast number of supplements and raw juices.

When we encouraged him to add oil and cooked food to his basically raw liquid food regime, he was more than doubtful. The idea of becoming fat and what people would think about him was terrifying. His overly concerns about what other people might think lead him to wrong decision making.

It was difficult to encourage him to listen to himself. What he thinks would be good as opposed to what people might think if he does something that he finds pleasurable, nourishing, soothing. He described his life as nothing less than paranoia. The paranoia of other people's opinion and criticism totally inhibited his life.

The more we heard the more we were concerned that the fences of his life that were originally there to protect him, had now changed into restricting him and taking away the joy of his life. Only when he indulged in cocaine binges, he felt that he got control over his life. He turned into the person he liked to be: cheerful, amusing and social.

During his treatments with abhyanga, shirodhara and therapeutic yoga though he discovered the more likable side of himself: subtle, gentle and warmhearted. He felt trust.

He said that he actually remembered himself being this person before his life took a hard turn and left him alone in pain and unpleasant memories. Feeling the gentleness and the ease again, he said, it was as if this person had been locked in. Stored somewhere.

His story was a story of fear and neglect from his early childhood. When his beloved parents divorced, he was sent to boarding school. His family wanted him to become something special, pure and religious and committed a terrible mistake: he and his younger brother were sent to a catholic boarding school, run by monks.

His first memories were those of sexual abuse and being forced to be silent about anything that happened. He said he lost his ability to cry in those years. He said, the wheezing started as he felt his body squashed under the body of an old monk. He could avoid sports, which meant changing clothes in change rooms due to his asthma. His health got fragile, deteriorated and by this helped him to escape at least some of the harassment and assaults.

Hay fever (V)

Atopic dermatitis on elbows and knees (V,P) No sports (K)

Alcoholic beverages like wine and beer, 3 portions in the evening (P) Suffers from sleeplessness, difficulties falling asleep, (V)

Day sleep (K)

Cocaine, (PV, tamas)

Amphetamin, (VP tamas)

Marijuana (K, tamas) Food choice:

Morning coffee with milk, müsli with milk and fruit (K;ama) In between: cheese sandwiches, creamy salads (KV, ama) Lunch: soup or food from nearby fast-food restaurants (ama) Snacks: ice cream, milk chocolate (ama, K)

Dinner: pizza or other delivery food, burger, pasta (KP, ama)

Digestion: 3-4 voluminous stools, smelly, oily, heavy (K,ama) Sweat profuse, smelly (P)

Urination: white (K)

No sex drive (VK)

Ayurvedic Consultation: V/K

Gunas R/T

Mamsa dhatu, medha dhatu, prana vaha srotas effected presence of ama.

Treatment:
Amapacana Pancakarma Herbs
Diet

Description And Result

Starting with vardhamana pippali for 13 days as a strict start to make him feel better rapidly. Though he felt insecure about our treatments, he wanted to give it a trial because his sleeplessness made him too fragile and suicidal at times.

He managed surprisingly quickly to change his bad dietary factors into no dairy, no fast food. Udvartana massages and steam bath to increase the feeling of his own body.

Followed by a long-term oileation massage series, twice a week. Each treatment was flanked with pranayama.

In the beginning, to deal with anger and sadness:

Kapalabhati

Combined with physical workout

After 3 weeks nadi shodhana and gentle introduction to relaxation methods like Jacobsen muscle relaxation method.

During his treatment, he was very easy to upset. His long-term hidden sadness, always covered by enormous stress and anger symptoms that he then suppressed with poor eating Of fatty, salty and sweet foods tried to make his way out.

We agreed not to let it out in cathartic procedures but instead allow the emotions to pass by and be observed.

Through gentle and calm observation of his state of mind, he was able to recognise when and how his breathing pattern changed, hardened and caused an onset of sinus blockage.

The change of eating habits was the most difficult part because his choice of fatty food gave him infantile stability and satisfaction.

Suppressing these urges caused an increase in blood pressure for a while.

We suggested again to do body work and introduced him to fast walking exercises. He started enjoying being in nature and a feeling of security was slowly growing.

Pancakarma

After 3 months of treatment, a Pancakarma Treatment was performed.

He went through heavy emesis, 5 times a day.

In the beginning, it was extremely difficult to touch his body below the navel, even on his lower back. Through applying massage with hot oil stamps he lost his discomfort quickly and loved it. Due to his former sexual abuse, we didn't perform basti, choosing haritaki in a little overdose instead.

He stopped smoking instantly with Pancakarma, felt as well much easier in keeping the new diet.

Sleep was improved from day one of Pancakarma.

No full set back of CRS or ARS ever since.

Treatment with herbs (what we get in the west)

Mustha churna 1/2 tsp before meals

Ashvagandha 1 tsp 3 times daily

Manasamitravatakam 2 tablets before bedtime

Triphala 1/2 tsp 3 times daily

Haritaki 2 Tabs, 2 times daily

Nasya with Anu Thail

Pranayama

So´Ham Chanting

Nadi shodhana 4-2-4-2 Shitali breathing and Brahmana humming.

Christina

Christina came to me on a recommendation by another singer. She was a singer, too, but she suffered from chronic sinus—rhinitis and bronchial asthma since she had moved to Germany from the US a couple of years ago. Her allergies stopped from singing most of the time. This seemed to me like a usual case and I thought that it would require mainly herbal treatment, which would fit into her tight budget plan.

She had mentioned that she had a tight budget when she set up the first appointment. The overall impression she made was a bit of a "hippie mum". Her very long hair was previously black but now greying, her jewellery was handmade of sparkling plastic beads, her scarfs were hand knitted. She came in with a guitar in one hand and one of her small children in the other hand, dressed in the same burgundy colours and hand knitted jumpers, a bit too big.

During the first consultation, she informed me that, besides her sinus problem, she also would like to have another baby. All of a sudden, the sinus problem seemed to be of minor interest.

She said that she was very short on money but she has heard that it is not a problem at my place and as soon as she would sing again, she could pay me or she would sing for me. I felt a bit run over. Her black eyes were sparkling and her face and that of her small child was firm with remarkably rosy cheeks. It was a cold Berlin winter day.

Christina explained to me that they are not used to central heating and that is why they are now brightly glowing in the warmth of the heated clinic room. It was one of the very long hour practice days when she arrived, snowing outside and I thought it could be a quick standard consultation. Interesting, too, as I had a number of patients suffering from CRS in that particular year.

(To explain the situation of allergies and the varieties in the city in each year, one has to understand Berlin. Berlin is a city of 4 million people, yet by law has to be covered by forest up to 47 per cent.

Berl.in is built in the middle of a swampy area, populated with the highest rate of wild animal species in Europe. Every year we face immigration of new plants like Ambrosia, a highly allergic weed, Solidago Virgoaurensis and others. Due to much warmer winters (from originally minus 23 degrees Celsius in January, February now to plus 10 degrees Celsius in the same months) weeds and trees are blossoming much earlier and each year different tree and weed pollen is dominant.

The previous raining season was June but now stretches from May till August, causing rotting of fruit and numerous insects to breed. Snowfalls are unpredictable till April and heavy storms are more frequent. Global climate changes are changing patient's complaints, too, in case of CRS, Allergies, Asthma, food intolerance, etc.)

So, I was interested in her allergy problems and had quickly agreed to see her for treating the sinus-rhinitis. Yet the child's wish was on a different page and the consultation then turned out being difficult as the focus kept on changing. While we were trying to analyse Christina's lifestyle, it turned out that there was more to discover and treat than a simple sinusitis that kept coming back.

She told me that they actually had no heating in the house since years. She explained, her husband was too old and fragile to look after the house or his family and she herself could not get the oven to work. They had no running water for a couple of days and the list of things that failed to work was growing. Her life was unexpectedly basic, with almost no such comfort of a modern life.

Her home was actually falling to pieces and everything seemed to be difficult to fix, even in a modern city. But it was a household of 3 little children and 2 adults. The place seemed to be in shambles. She seemed to ignore this as much as she asked for compassion for her situation in a contradicting manner.

By giving the idea that everything was under control and a new baby would complete her life, however, at the same time she allowed us to see her life as a patchwork of dysfunctional household, relationships and no earnings. She returned to the focus again and again on her future pregnancies as well as on the mourning of her last 4 miscarriages whenever we tried to emphasise that the obvious problems should be fixed first.

A total number of eight pregnancies that ended sadly in miscarriages and a forced abortion would have been enough to traumatise a woman and leave her with anxiety of more losses. Christina made one believe that she would be the woman who wanted nothing more but being a loving mother and a part-time artist.

At the same time, she appeared to be a helpless mother, overwhelmed by difficulties and who does not act responsible for her children. Being financially broke in an insecure place with small children and a husband who could barely look after himself, she was determined to have even more children. Besides the unknown underlying medical condition that led to the miscarriages, her husband was not even willing to have more children. However, a pathological reasoning might drive and motivate her to actually ignore her own needs—and those of her children—for security and health.

She reported that she had lost her appetite recently. Cooking for herself, the children or her husband was only occasional. She mentioned being very much underweight (V) for years but now started "feeling really fat". She actually was very lean with wider hips. She tried to explain her chronic feeling of no appetite now and the feeling of no appetite in her childhood and teens—there seemed to be a link that she denied. As a child and teenager, no one cared about her losing weight to a degree where it even became risky and she was considered 30% underweight.

Now, in her marriage, her husband widely ignored her. He seemed not to care if she lost or gained weight. He seemed to have enough of her. Her cry for help by not feeding herself was not heard. The question came up: was there any connection to her miscarriages? As underweight causes a decrease in female hormones as well as nutritional sources for the unborn, a mother that starves herself does not prepare herself for a long journey. The baby is already at risk. The unborn is becoming a victim by her mother, who seeks to be nurtured but ignores the needs of the growing life inside her.

Traumatised people tend to repeat their pain and trauma unconsciously.

What could have been Christina's experience? Why she wanted to risk so much? Why was she unable to care for herself and, by not knowing her own needs, could not respond to the needs of others?

After a couple of treatments with pranayama and careful education in ayurveda nutrition and herbal therapy with selected Medhya Rasayanas, she felt safe enough to open up her past.

Painfully, she remembered being raped repeatedly by her own uncle at the family home starting at the age of 12. An abortion was forced on her, although she said she wanted to keep the baby as it was a part of her that they wanted to pull out of her. A midwife then injected toxic substances, including cleaning products, into her uterus. Getting pregnant significantly showed her victory over the violence of the family, yet the miscarriages kept on repeating the unsolved trauma of loss. The child she wanted to bear was almost an image of her own inner child, repeatedly failing to protect it.

When she came for treatments or check-ups, she always was a bit overly charming and persuasive, so a medical communication was difficult. I always felt like in some ping-pong match, where we both tried to make a point and win. If I did not agree to what she was convinced of, she got easily argumentative and irritable, ready to leave. I redirected the consultations therefore into written home works and lists of things to be done and remembered. A daily text message confirmed that she had done what she was asked to change in her lifestyle.

As Christina had completed a list of her food, drinks and lifestyle (Ahara/Vihara) it became obvious that she had an alcohol problem. It was something not to give up easily despite her wanting to be pregnant. The dulling moments of wine in the evenings were sadly needed. Yet an admitted average of half a bottle of wine was definitely too risky for an unborn child.

However, she followed closely the herbal treatments and the instructed breathing exercises. Christina's chronic sinus infection subsided very quickly through the breathing and herbal treatment and though did the asthma after her house got a good clean. She obviously suffered from the constant dust and concrete exposure. The restauration of the heating helped as well. She got pregnant after 6 months and was overly excited and not worried because she had decided to leave all responsibility to me (which I never ever would have offered!).

It is definitely not the goal of any treatment that the patient claims that the therapist is from now on responsible for everything after.

Thankfully, after 9 months she gave birth to a healthy baby girl, weighing 4 kg.

At this time, she still maintained to her routine of 1-2 glasses of wine daily.

She was a patient that was so difficult to handle. Like mercury, one could not get hold of her inner being. Although her overall charming nature and her ideas of simplicity and living in nature were all appealing. But she was narcissistic, manipulative, irritable and became easily unpleasant. She made all sensible interventions a real struggle.

I remembered the first days of my education in ayurveda where Professor S.N.Gupta from Nadiad, Gujarat, quoted Charaka, saying, one should not treat the patient who is poor, does not listen or has no compliance (In his own words: *Don't treat the naughty patient*).

I always felt that I have to make it work somehow. This is a problem in my own biography. In Christina's case I realised that the patient who is mentally disturbed (*unmada*) with a borderline syndrome like in Christina's case could be ready to harm herself, others or the doctor.

Charkas rules explain why we should not treat the "naughty" patient:

There might be no success in the treatment or the treatment itself could harm the patient as it might not be completed, interrupted or wrongly misused.

Mental disturbances can easily lead to further wrong assumptions and actions.

I was concerned about her as I have had so much to struggle in the consultations to keep the right balance that is needed for a sensible treatment. I started feeling resistance for setting up appointments, I felt avoidance pattern coming up in myself as I tried to keep calm during all the manipulative speech. The sweet-sounding persuasiveness of her also affected my clinic staff.

When she tried to convince me to do certain things or agree to her and I insisted on the plan, she went to my staff and complained about me being hard, incompetent or heartless. They did not realise the manipulation and then happily did everything that I had not agreed to or even came up to me to tell me off. After she had her baby, she then left, leaving only a quick text message. And we all went back to normal.

After 2 years, though, she came back, now at the age of 45, saying she is now ready for another baby, although her husband strongly objects to it.

We sat down and we tried to breathe through the feeling of the moments she actually spent with her 4 children.

She realised that she was actually avoiding intimacy. By having another baby, she would have been busy again with the needs of a newborn, where she can be dominant. Dealing with growing up children though is different. One has to listen, communicate, relate and allow oneself to be present in this moment. Christina said that this rang a bell and she wants to explore this feeling, wants to give it a chance—

It is often extremely difficult for traumatised people to allow intimacy. Their partners and children, all suffer from the feeling that they are not enough, that they are unwanted, just because the traumatised patient is cut off from her feelings. Her inability to express feelings of intimacy, closeness, her lack of ability to care and be responsible reflects on the children. Generations of traumatised families unfortunately reproduce the patterns of pain, neglect and loneliness.

I recently heard from her and she said she had decided not to have another child.

Treatment:

Reconstructing the home

Following a proper dinacharya

pranayama, in the clinic and as homework, nadi shodhana, daily, kapalabhati

+Medication: dravyaguna:

Mustha 1/4 tsp-1/4 tsp-1/4 Tsp

Manjishtha 1/4 Tsp-0-1/4 Tsp

Guduci 1/4 Tsp-0-1/4 Tsp

No coffee, reduction of alcohol, proper sleep and eating times

Thoughts after 40 years of practice –

As I sat down after the years of writing and needed to decide what to share with the public and I realised how important it is to guide and teach young colleagues in the alternative or complementary field of healing about traumatic injuries. In the recent years, people got more interested and many courses for trauma—sensitive yoga or other disciplines appeared.

However they might help the traumatised patient, they never addressed the therapist, the yoga teacher, the acupuncturist or ayurvedic practitioner themselves. Neither did they inform them how to protect oneself nor did they offer learning and supervising the young therapist. All of them are so enthusiastic about healing and trauma became almost a mainstream event that everyone obviously went through and wanted to heal from.

Many of us have lived through trauma, are survivors of domestic abuse, of racial assault, have lived through stressful and painful periods in our lives and have or haven't healed. However, many of us are also driven by a narcissistic personality disorder that needs attention and who might give more attention and adoration than most of the traumatised patients?

Creating abusive relationships between therapists and patients is one part of the same picture that we should not oversee but speak out loud. This is not limited to cults and sexual abusive relationships between the person who offers "healing" from trauma, but also to reckless money making or unclear boundaries that stop the patient from recovery and only serves the "healer", "therapist" or whatever they might call themselves.

As mentioned earlier in this book, people with an imprint of DA (domestic abuse), a history of child abuse or other unfortunately got "trained" to choose devaluating relationships on all levels. They keep still, they even might adore the predator. Many of us are working in the field of medicine as we like to help, we like to maybe please people, we like to be in control. That could display our own trauma background and when we look at statistics, there is an unproportionally high number of traumatised people actually working as helpers, nurses, doctors, social workers, alternative healers, yoga teachers, ayurvedic therapists and so on.

Most of the trauma patients are kind and helpful and compliant. They want to integrate their ugly and painful haunting experiences in their life's narrative so they can sleep at night and live in the present.

But there are the others, who's traumatic experiences have changed their nature into a person that is able to harm, to assault, disrespect, manipulate or traumatise us.

It was more than once that I got attacked by survivors who were waiting for me outside, forced themselves into the practice when they thought I was alone, who were terrorising me with phone calls and threats of all kinds. Luckily I was not harmed but I changed habits and became more cautious and that is another reason why I wrote this book. I wanted to give students and health workers the tools at their hands to recognise a traumatised patient and to develop a sense for their predictable actions according to the ayurveda concepts of the doshas and the gunas.

I strongly emphasise that we all get a good supervision on our work. On our partnerships. Our relationships. On our relation to the world.

We need not only sensible education in Ayurveda Psychiatry, Western Psychiatry and all the ancient and recent scientific studies but a network for the supervision of all therapists for the safety of our patients as for own safety and healing and progress in the field of understanding trauma as well as recovery from trauma.

And in this book, I hope I have taken you on my very personal story and journey of inquiry of the understanding of recovery through meaning making. Meaning making became the most significant " side effect" of all the treatments that I and my team have enrolled. It was nothing that we taught the patient, we never emphasised on any result or belief that people should adapt in order to heal. so all the meaning making was truly their own experience, their own inner journey and differed from one patient to the other.

I remember one patient who was shattered from her life experiences and came to us on a day when she felt: it is enough, I cannot go through this anymore, I want to die. She came to us, determined to commit suicide if the treatment won' t help NOW. She asked me: what's the meaning in life? And honestly spoken, I suddenly had absolutely no idea what to say! I could not make up a meaning.

At the same time, I felt life being so fragile, vanishing within seconds and taking for granted at the same time. Cancer patients who struggle to survive had sometimes a past of suicidal attempts, people, who could look back to a satisfying and lavish lifestyle felt emptiness and loneliness within their relationships and could not see any meaning in life. A purpose, a meaning, was this necessary?

If exactly this meaning or purpose could be shattered by events like leaving the country after having lost all belongings in a war, after losing health or family members, was this meaning, purpose the core of the existence ? And is it the ultimate truth for everyone? What is it that shapes us and what is it that creates resilience?

But over the years, I had become a witness to the arising of meaning that was different from purpose. And even different from meaning in its very sense. The meaning dissolved into the word of "Dharma". We, patients, therapists, me, started to think outside the box. One of the popular boxes is "Karma".

From there we move on into the legacy of Dharma, meaning, away from action-reaction, back to what is it to be human? Finding emotions and feelings that unfold like kindness, empathy, serenity and happiness. Finding the connection. In my eyes, the human connection through kindness is the happiness that we were looking for. Through the experiences during the ayurveda and yoga Therapy treatments with pranayama, patients were able to experience this beautiful state of mind on their inner journey.

In this, I am so grateful to all my teachers and guides who trustfully opened up their treasure box of wisdom so we can connect and heal.

Dr Anastasia Shchedrina:

Manuela has always taught me to be curious. Her interests are extremely broad and she is open to everything—that is, everything which she can use to help her patients. She has been active in the field of naturopathy for more than 40 years.

This book embodies Manuela's professional journey as a naturopathy practitioner, conceptualised through an academic, scientific lens. For the past years, ayurveda and yoga have been the main systems within which Manuela has been working; she has chosen to treat trauma and PTSD using the two systems. Ayurveda puts much emphasis on the need for balance and her book is also about balance between western and Eastern medical systems; between science and intuition; between critical thinking and faith.

Manuela herself admits to being of mixed descent, as well as to having been connected to Asia since her childhood. This is clearly reflected in her book, as she treats yoga and ayurveda with great respect, avoiding both the western colonial approach and an unreasonable fascination for the two systems.

Manuela's book discusses the phenomenon of trauma and PTSD as well as standard psychotherapy methods from unexpected angles. For instance, she uses her own example to illustrate that trauma may result in a seemingly 'normal' behaviour such as an ideally clean house or any other type of extreme perfectionism—something to which the western therapeutic school pays little attention.

Of great interest are her reflections on memory and reminiscences, e.g., on how patients get tired of having to turn to their reminiscences frequently. Thus, the corporal approaches and the ancient knowledge offered by ayurveda and yoga can prove highly effective in treating trauma and handling PTSD.

The classification of stages of PTSD based on the doshas and gunas dominant at each stage, along with the ensuing therapeutic recommendations, has particularly fascinated me, as this is the first time I encounter such an approach. Notably, these are not mere ideas or hypotheses—these are the results of Manuela's extensive empirical research.

The author pays particular attention to the issues facing women in modern society, including the violence they have to endure—something that is still frequently silenced. Most notably, Manuela always respects her patients' cultural identities and backgrounds and she considers those factors during therapy. Of course, this has been reflected in the book as well.

Detailed descriptions of yoga breathing exercises and ayurvedic procedures showcase the author's professionalism, but they also speak volumes about how she has been transferring the knowledge provided under the two Indian systems into the western one.

The book will be of interest to a wide range of readers because it significantly broadens one's perceptions of trauma and PTSD, providing unexpected perspectives on those issues. Therapists will be interested in this book because it gives an account of the author's unique, years-long experience in naturopathy, conceptualised academically within the context of the western medicine.

As for me, I am endlessly grateful for having Manuela in my life; for the many years of joint work; for the fact that she has become my friend and mentor; for how she discovers the untapped potential in her friends and colleagues and helps them harness it. We have been working together for many years now and I still learn something new from Manuela—not just in terms of ayurveda, but also in terms of the sheer curiosity about the various aspects of life, the desire to try them out—and then to offer the best to patients!

Literature:

Avery, T. J. (2018) 'Yoga and PTBS: A Primer on Symptoms and Potential Mechanisms of Change', *Yoga Therapy Today (YTT)*, International Association of Yoga Therapists, Winter, p14-16.

Behere, P. a.o. (2018) *Ayurvedic concepts related to psychotherapy*, http://www.indianjpsychiatry.org, IP: [62.182.203.157], seen 16.07.2020. https://www.britannica.com/science/Ayurveda, seen on 07.08.2020.

Bhusal, N., *Shirodhara in the management of chittodvegajanya anindra* (insomnia due to generalised anxiety disorder) https://www.allresearchjournal.com/archives/2017/vol3issue8/PartC/3-8-32-134.pdf, seen 09.09.20

Bmfsfj, *Murderer in Relationsships: Zu den Morden an Frauen in der Partnerschaft*, https://www.bmfsfj.de/bmfsfj/aktuelles/presse/pressemitteilungen/gewalt-gegen-frauen---zahlen-weiterhin-hoch-ministerin-giffey-startet-initiative--staerker-als-gewalt-/141688, seen 13.06.20.

Bose, B. and Tripathy, D. (2013) 'Secondary metabolite profiling, cytotoxicity, anti-inflammatory potential and in-vitro inhibitory activities of Nardostachys jatamansi on key enzymes linked to hyperglycemia, hypertension and cognitive disorders', PMID 30668444,DOI 10.1016/j.phymed.2018.08.010, *Indian Psychiatry*, 55(Suppl 2):S310-314.Doi:10.4103/0019-5545.105556.

Charakasamhitahotline, (2020) *Behavioural and Psychological Manifestation of Triguna*, http:// Charakasamhitaonline.com/mediawiki, p 10 of 12, seen 20.08.2020

Choudry, B. (MD, PhD.) (2015) 'Approach to Neurological Disorder in Ayurveda', *Indian Journal of Medical Research and Pharmaceutical Sciences*, ISSN 2349-5340

Compson, A. (2010) 'Insanity: Ayurvedic vs. Western Medicine Perspectives', *California Institute for Ayurveda*, US, https://www.ayurvedacollege.com/blog/insanity/, seen 12.3.20.

Yogi Coudoux (2004) *Breathing Life*, Mumbai (Indian Edition): Embassy Book Distributors, ISBN 978-81-88452-37-8

Cousins, R. (2018) 'A Quarterly Technical Assistance Journal on Disaster Behavioural Health, Samhsa', *Disaster Technical Assistance centre*, Vol 14, Issue 1, US, seen 7/2020, https://www.samhsa.gov/sites/default/files/dtac/dialogue-volis1_final_051718.pdf.

Damasio, A. (2019) *The Strange order of Things, Life, Feeling and the Making of Cultures,* New York: Penguin Press, 1. Edition, ISBN 978-0-307-90876-6 Vintage Books.

Desikachar, T. K. V. (2006) *Reflections on Yoga Sutras of Patanjali* (Paperback for Sale in India only), Chennai-35: Quadra Press Ltd., 2nd Reprint.

Edel, H. (1999) *Atemtherapie*, München: Urban und Fischer, Jena, 6.Auflage, 3.edition, ISBN 3-437-46480-9.

Ekman, Weidenfeld and Nicolson (2019) *Emotions revealed*, ISBN 978-0-7538-1765-0, UK.

Elz, J. **Verurteilungsquoten und Einstellungsgründe**, Was wissen wir wirklich? KRIMZ: Kriminologische Zentralstelle, pp. 117-141, https://www.krimz.de/fileadmin/dateiablage/E-Publikationen/KUP72-Elz.pdf, seen on 25.04.19)

Emerson, David, Hopper and Elizabeth (2014) *Trauma-Yoga*, Heilung durch sorgsame Körperarbeit, Probst Verlag, Lichtenau/Westfalen 2012,2.Auflage 2014, ISBN 978-3-9813389-4-2

England, D. (2017) *Soulfulness, Soulfulness*, London (UK): Karnac Books, 1.edition, ISBN 978-1-78220-475-6.

'Violence against Women—an EU-wide Survey', *European Union Agency for Fundamental Rights*, https://fra.europa.eu/en/publication/2014/violence-against-women-eu-wide-survey-main-results-report, seen 14.10.2019

Frazzetto, G. (2013) *How we feel, What Neuroscience can-and can't tell us about our emotions Doubleday,* UK: Transworld Publishers, ISBN 9780857521248.

Gandhi, S. and Wolff, L. (2017) *Yoga and the Roots of Cultural Appropriation, Art, Music and Pop Culture,* https://www.kzoo.edu/praxis/yoga/ seen 6/2020

Goulston, M. (M.D.) (2008) *Post-Traumatic Stress Disorder for Dummies*, ISBN 978-0-470-4922-8

Government US (2018) *How common is PTSD in Veterans?,* www.ptsd.va.gov/understand/common/common_veterans.asp, seen 27.07.20.

Graham, C. L. (2010) *Happiness Around the World: The Paradox of Happy Peasants and Miserable Millionaires,* DOI:

10.1093/acprof:osobl/9780199549054.001.0001, ISBN 9780199549054.

Gupta, S. N. and Stapelfeldt, E. (2019) *Ayurveda Medizin*, 3. Auflage, ISBN 9783132421981.

Haines, S. *Trauma is Really Strange*, UK: Singing Dragon Publications, ISBN 978-1-84-819-293-5.

Härle, D. (2013) *Körperorientierte Traumatherapie*, Dagmar Härle, Paderborn: Junfermann Verlag, ISBN 978-3-95571-333-1.

van der Hart, O. (2008) *Das verfolgte Selbst* (The Haunted Self), Paderborn: Junfermann Verlag, ISBN 978-3-87387-671-2.

Jacobsen, M. (2002) **Prakriti in Shamkhya-Yoga**, *Material Principle, Religious Experience, Ethical Implications*, Delhi: Banarassidass, , ISBN 81-208-1827-x, Indian subcontinent only, 1. Indian edition.

Jeffreys, M. (M.D.) *PTSD: National Centre for PTSD, Clinician s Guide to Medications for PTSD*,
https://www.ptsd.va.gov/professional/treat/txessentials/clinician_guide_meds.a sp, Seen 23.12.2019.

Kapfhammer, K. (Prof. Dr) **Trauma und Traumafolgestörungen**, Österreichische Gesellschaft für Neuropsychopharmakologie und Biologische Psychiatrie,seen 7/2020
https://oegpb.at/2018/05/28trauma-und-traumafolgestörungen/

Kelly (2013) *Integrated Treatment of Substance Use and Psychiatric Disorders*,
https://www.ncbi.nlm.nih.gov/pmc/articles/PMC3753025/, seen 4/2020.

Van der Kolk, Bessel, Publications
https://www.besselvanderkolk.com/resources/scientific-publications since 1984
Post-traumatic stress Disorder, 1987, Psychological Trauma, seen 20.10.2020

Van der Kolk, Bessel, **Verkörperter Schrecken, Traumaspuren in Gehirn, Geist und Körper und wie man sie heilen kann** (The Body keeps the Score, Original Titel) Probst Verlag, Lichtenau, Westfalen, 2015, ISBN 978-3-944476-13-1

KriPoz, **Entschädigung:** Staatliche Opferentschädigung und Adhäsionsverfahren Reformbedarf in

Deutschlandhttps://kripoz.de/2018/05/28/staatliche-opferentschaedigung-und-adhaesionsverfahren-reformbedarf-in-deutschland-und-china/ (Compensation for Victims of Terror attacks, sexual abuse and others in Germany and China),20.09.20

Kundu, C. a.o. other, *The Role of Psychic Factors in Pathogenesis of Essential Hypertension and It's Management by Shirodhara and Sarpagandha Vati*, Pub Med, PMID 22048535 https://pubmed.ncbi.nlm.nih.gov/22048535/ 12.04.20.

Lad, V. (2015) *Ayurvedic Perspectives on Selected Pathologies*, 3rd Edition, The Ayurvedic Institute, ISBN 978-1-883725-24-2.

Lavekar, G. (Dr) *Glimpse of Mental Disorders and Treatment in Ayurveda*, CCRAS-AYUSHM Govt. of India, Ayurvedasept2013Lavekarspage.pdf.

Lee (2017) *Beyond Drugs, the Universal Experience of Addiction,* Source:https,://drgabormate.com/opioids-universal-experience-addiction/ seen 25.07.20.

Levine, P. *Case Studies,* https://www.psychalive.org/video-dr-peter-levine-on-somatic-experiencing-ptsd/seen 16.8.20.

Levine, P. (PhD) (2010) *In An Unspoken Voice*, Berkeley California: North Atlantic Books, ISBN 078-1-55643-943-8.

Levine, P. A. (PhD) (2015) *Trauma and Memory*, Berkeley California: North Atlantic Books, ISBN 978-1-58394-994-8.

Lingham, D. (Rodney) (2015) *Aushad Rahasya, The Secret of Ayurvedic Herbs and Disorders of the Mind,* revised edition, New Zealand: Lulu.com, ISBN 978-1-304-08378-4.

Liu,Prf.,Schiemann, Prof. **Staatliche Opferentschädigung und Adhäsionsverfahren Reformbedarf in Deutschland und China,** KriPoz, Kriminalpolitische Zeitschrift, Prof.Liu,Prf.Schiemann,pdf.5/2020 https://kripoz.de/2018/05/28/staatliche-opferentschaedigung-und-adhaesionsverfahren-reformbedarf-in-deutschland-und-china/ Seen, 12.12.20

Lobo, Roque, **Diagnosisverfahren zur Feststellung, ob Probanden unter Streß leiden und ob Geräte oder Arbeitsplätze ergonomisch gerecht gestaltet sind, Rocque Lobo,**

1997https://patents.google.com/patent/DE19734918A1/de, seen 23.10.2020

Marques, D. *What makes people happy around the world/ art and culture*, https://www.happiness.com/en/magazine/art-culture-leisure/what-makes-people-happy-happiness-in-different-cultures/2020, seen 05.04.20.

McMackin, R. A. and McMackin (Ed) *Trauma Therapy in Context: the Science and Craft of Evidence-based Practise*, ISBN-13:978-1-4338-2,2012.

Malhotra, R., Manohar, R. (Prof.) (2020) *Dosha= Humour, Infinity foundation*.

Mana, F. (2013) *Breathing techniques for free-diving*, Magenes, 2. Edition, Magenes editorial.

Manohar, Ram (Prof.) (2019) *Ayurvedic Psychology*, PowerPoint Presentation at REAA 2019.

Manohar, R. (Prof.) (2018) *Indian Psychology—An Ayurvedic Perspective* (Part 1 and 2), Centre for IndicStudies, https://www.youtube.com/results?search_query=ram+manohar+indic+studies.

Mate, G. (MD) (2010) *In the Realm of the Hungry Ghosts*, North Atlantic Books, ISBN 978-1-55643-880-6.

Masic, I. (2014) *Ethics in Medical Research*, https://www.ncbi.nlm.nih.gov/pmc/articles/PMC4192767, PMCID: PMC4192767.

Mate, G. (2013) *The Power of Addiction, The Addiction to Power*, Ted Conference, Ted x Rio, YouTube, https://www.youtube.com/results?search_query=the+power+of+addiction+gab or, seen 21.08.20.

Mate, G. (M.D.) (2011) *When the Body says No, Exploring the Stress-Disease Connection,* Hoboken (New Jersey): John Wiley and Sons Inc, ISBN 978 0 471 21982 8.

Ministerium für Familie, Senioren, Frauen und Jugend, **Gewalt gegen Frauen**, 2019,https://www.bmfsfj.de/bmfsfj/aktuelles/presse/pressemitteilungen/gewalt-gegen-frauen---zahlen-weiterhin-hoch-ministerin-giffey-startet-initiative--staerker-als-gewalt-/141688, seen 13.11.2020

(Minkoff, 2001, PTSD and Substance Use Disorder Comorbidity Treatment, p. 273)

Mitscherlich, Alexander u. Margarete, **Die Unfähigkeit zu trauern,** Grundlagen kollektiven Verhaltens, Mitscherlich, Piper and Co. Verlag, ISBN 3-492-00468-7, München, 1977

Mittwede, M. (Prof.) (1998) *Der Ayurveda*, Heidelberg: Haug Verlag, ISBN 3-7760-1654-x.

Dr Murthy, A. R. V, (2004) *The Mind in Ayurveda and other Indian Traditions*, Delhi: Chaukambha Sanskrit Pratishtan, ISBN 81-7084-272-2.

Nachtomy, O. and Shifroni, E. (2019) *The Psycho-physical Lab, Yoga practice and the Mind-Body Problem*, Mudita Books, Amazon Distribution, ISBN 978 965 9251964.

Najavits, L. (2012) *Posttraumatic Stress Disorder and Substance use Disorder Comorbidity Treatment: Principles and Practices in Real World Settings*, https://psycnet.apa.org/record/2011-29969-013, seen 13.04.2020.

Nemetchek, M. (2016) *The Ayurvedic plant Bacopa monnieri inhibits inflammatory pathways in the brain*, Elsevier Ireland Ltd., free PMC, PMID: 27473605, DOI: 10.1016/j.jep.2016.07.073, https://www.ncbi.nlm.nih.gov/pmc/articles/PMC5269610/ seen 12.12.20.

Nestor, J. (2020) *Breath: The New Science of a Lost Art*, UK: Penguin life, ISBN 9780241289075.

Nuernberger, P. (PhD.) (1981) *Freedom from Stress*, Himalayan International Institute of Yoga Science and Philosophy of the USA, ISBN 0-89389-064-2.

Ogden, P. and Minton, K. (2010) *Trauma und Körper*, Paderborn: Junfermann Verlag, ISBN 978—3—87387—717—7.

Pelizzari, U. and Tovaglieri, S. (2004) *Manuel of Free-diving, Underwater on a single breath*, Reddick (USA), ISBN 19286649270.

Porkert, M. (Prof.) (1996) *Die Chinesische Medizin,* Düsseldorf: Econ Verlag, ISBN 9-783612204202.

Pratte, M. and Nanavastti, K. a.o. (2017) *An alternative treatment for anxiety: a systematic review of human trial results reported for the Ayurvedic herb ashvagandha (Withania somnifera),* 197:92-100.doi 10.1016/j.jep.2016.07.03. Epub 2016 jul26PMID25405876, seen 16.07.2020.

Swami Rama and Ballantine, R. (MD) (2014) *Yoga and Psychotherapy: The Evolution of Consciousness*, Allahabad (India): Himalaya Institute Publications, ISBN 13-978-089389-036-0.

Rastogi, S. (ed.) a.o. (2014) *Ayurvedic Science of Food and Nutrition*, London: Springer Verlag, Heidelberg, ISBN 978-1-4614-9628-1.

Rhyner, H. (2004) *Das neue Ayurveda Praxisbuch*, Urania, Neuhausen/Schweiz, ISBN 3-03819-049-7.

Roberts, A. L. (Psychol. Med.) (2011) *Race/ethnic differences in exposure to traumatic events, development of post-traumatic stress disorder and treatment-seeking for post-traumatic stress disorder in the United States*, 41(1): 71-83.

Published online 29 Mar 2010, doi: 10.1017/S0033291710000401, seen 01.12.20.

Robila, M. (2018) *Refugees and Social Integration in Europe*, United Nations Department of Economic and Social Affairs (UNDESA) Division for Social Policy and Development, United Nations Expert Group Meeting, New York, https://www.un.org/development/desa/family/wp-content/uploads/sites/23/2018/05/Robila_EGM_2018.pdf, seen 06.12.20.

Rothenberg, R. L. (2020) *Restoring Prana*, London/Philadelphia: Singing Dragon Publications, ISBN 978-1-84819-401-4.

Rosen, R. (2002) *The Yoga of Breath*, Boston/London: Shambala Publications, ISBN 978-1-57062-889-4.

Saraswati, S. N.(2011) *Mind, Mind Management and Raja Yoga*, Bihar (India): Yoga Publication Trust Munger.

Satyananda, S. and Yoga, V. (2007) *A Systematic Course in the Ancient Tantric Techniques of Yoga and Kriya*, India: Yoga Publication Trust, ISBN 8185787085.

Schmidbauer, W. (2018) *Die Geheimnisse der Kränkung und das Rätsel des Narzissmus*, Stuttgart: Klett Cotta, ISBN9783-608-89230-7.

Schnyder, U. (2013) *Trauma und Schmerz*, Bonn: Schattauer Verlag, ISBN 978-3-7945-2892-9.

Scott et al., (2013) *Associations between Lifetime Traumatic Events and Subsequent Chronic Physical Conditions: A Cross-National, Cross-Sectional Study,*
https://journals.plos.org/plosone/article?id=10.1371/journal.pone.0080573, seen 2020/8.

Sharma, P. V., **(1999)** *Sushrut, Sushrut-Samhita* with English translation of text and Dalhana's commentary along with critical notes Vol.-1, first Edition, Varanasi (India): Chaukhambha Vishvabharati.

Dr Shastri, A. (2001) *Sushruta, Sushruta-Samhita* along with Ayurveda-Tattvasandipika Hindi Vyakhya Part-1, Varanasi (India): Chaukhambha Sanskrit Sansthan, 12. edition.

Sepahvand, A. *On Faggot Translation,* Ruskin School of Art.

St John's College, University of Oxford, Paper for Transfer of Status from Probationary Researcher to D.Phil (Fine Art Practice) October 5, 2020

Sen-Gupta, O. (2017) *Im Herz des Yoga Übens*, 1. Edition, Original title: The Heart of Practice, Understanding Yoga from Inside, tao.de Verlag, Bielefeld, ISBN 978-3-96051-793-1.

Sharma, A. K. and Gupta, R. (2003) *Role of Shirodhara in the Management of Anidra (Insomnia) and Chittovega (Anxiety Neurosis):* A Clinical Study, (received all 6-2-03) JR.A.S.Vol.XXIV, No.3-4, pp 104-113.

Sharma, R. K. and Dash, B. (2000) *Charaka Samhita*, Vol. I-III, Varanasi (India): Chowkhamba Sanskrit Series Office, ISBN 81-7080-013-7, 6. Edition.

Dr Shaw, J. (2018) *Böse: Making Evil*, Hanser Verlag, München 1. Auflage, deutsch, ISBN 978-3-446-26029-0.

Shaw, J. (MD) (2019) *Making Evil, The Science behind Humanity's Dark Side*, UK: Canongate Books, ISBN 978—1—78689—130—3.

Shaw, J. (MD) (2016) *The Memory Illusion, The Science of False Memory,* London (UK): Random House Books, ISBN 978—1847—9476—11.

Acharya Shrinivasa, G. (Dr) (2009) *Panchakarma Illustrated,* Delhi (India): Chaukhamba Sanskrit Pratishthan, reprint 2009, ISBN 8170843079.

S2k—Leitlinie: Diagnostik und Behandlung von akuten Folgen psychischer Traumatisierung,Juli 2019,AWMF online, seen 9/2019

Skuban, R. *Pranayama, Die heilsame Kraft des Atems,* Aquamarin Verlag,3. Auflage, Grafing, ISBN 978-3-89427-793-2.

Solomon, P. (1961) *Sensory deprivation*: a symposium held at Harvard Medical School, 1961 https://psycnet.apa.org/record/1961-35085-000, seen 4/19.

Steer, E. (2017) 'A Cross comparison between Ayurvedic etiology of Major Depressive Disorder and bidirectional effect on gut dysregulation', *Journal of Ayurveda and Integrative Medicine (J-AIM)*, USA: Teachers College Columbia, published online 2019.

Steger, M. and Park, C. (2012) *The creation of meaning following trauma: Meaning making and trajectories of distress and recovery,* https://psycnet.apa.org/record/2011-29969-008, seen 8/19.

Stephens, M. (2017) *Yoga Therapy, Foundations, Methods and Practices for Common Ailments*, Berkeley California: North Atlantic Books, ISBN 97—81623171063.

Sutton, N. (2017) *The Yoga Sutras of Patanjali*, Oxford Centre of Hindu Studies, ISBN 978-1-5272-10-37-0.

Thompson, D. (1999) *The Ayurvedic Diet*: *The Ancient Way to Health Rejuvenation and Weight Control*, New Delhi (India): New Age Books, ISBN 978-81-7822-014-7.

Tiwari, M. (2010) *Ayurveda: A Life of Balance*, Delhi: Motilal Banarsidass, reprint 2010, Indian Edition, ISBN 978-81208-2076-2.

US military, *Demographic of US Military*, www.cfr.org/backgrounder/demographics-us-military, 20.8.2020, seen 5/2020.

Voss, J. (2018) *Meaning in Life*, *Springer Nature*, London (UK): Macmillan Publishers, ISBN 978-1-137-57668-2.

Valiathan, M. S.(2009) *The Legacy of Charaka*, Universities Press (India) Private Limited 2009, reprinted 2011, ISBN 978-81-7371-667-6.

Verma, V. (1995) *Ayurveda-a Way of Life*, York Beach (Maine): Samuel Weiser Inc., ISBN 0-87728-822-4.

Vinjamuri, S. a.o. (2011) 'Pancakarma Ayurvedic Detoxification and Allied Therapies-Is there any Evidence?', *Evidence based Practice in Complementary and Alternative Medicine*, pp 113-137, http://link-springer-com-443.webvpn.fjmu.edu.cn/chapter/10.1007%2F978-3-642-24565-7_7.

Wittgenstein, L. (1979) 'Tractatus logicus philosophicus', *Logisch-Philosophische Abhandlung*, Edition suhrkamp12, 14. edition, Germany: Suhrkamp Verlag.

Dr Yadav, S. (2015) *Concept of Shat-Kriya-Kala*, https://www.boloji.com/articles/48760/concept-of-shat-kriya-kala

Swami Yogakanti (2007) **Sanskrit Glossary of Yogic terms**, Yoga Publication Trust, Bihar School of Yoga ; Mungar, Bihar, India, ISBN 978 8186336311.

www.ingramcontent.com/pod-product-compliance
Lightning Source LLC
Chambersburg PA
CBHW040107180526
45172CB00009B/1254